PRAISE FOR *EAT TO LOVE*

"This is not your traditional nutrition book. It is political, scientific, and spiritual. It is all encompassing—mind, body, and soul. *Eat to Love* teaches you to create space through meditation and find your daily practice of nourishing yourself inside-out."

LAURA CIPULLO, RD, CDE, CEDRD, RYT; founder of L'ifestyle Lounge and immediate past president of IAEDP NY

"*Eat to Love* is a roadmap to finding our way home to our body and developing a more peaceful, loving, and compassionate relationship with food, our body, and our selves. Jenna Hollenstein combines her extensive nutrition expertise as a registered dietitian with Buddhist principles to help readers resolve their eating issues through a spiritual lens. She manages to make it easily digestible for readers who are new to Buddhist philosophy while also stimulating more experienced practitioners. I can't recommend this book highly enough!"

ALEXIS CONASON, PsyD, clinical psychologist, and founder of the Anti-Diet Plan

"No more neglecting the intelligence of our bodies, let *Eat to Love* bring nourishing ourselves back to our naturally smart, trustworthy, intuitive selves!"

EMME, TV host and body image advocate (@supermodelemme)

"If you want to develop a deeper understanding around your food and body challenges, read *Eat to Love*. But if you want to revolutionize the way you relate to food and body image then I invite you to pore over the pages of Jenna's book. With profound insight, expertise, and tangible tools, Jenna provides the most complete guide to help you find greater peace with food and body. I cannot recommend this book more highly."

MARCI EVANS, MS, CEDRD-S, LDN, CPT

"*Eat to Love* is a book to help you get bigger: a bigger heart, a bigger understanding of why you eat, and a bigger sense of gratitude for your body. Too often, during the act of dieting these senses are lost, and for individuals who are experts at dieting, this necessary awareness may have been forgotten. *Eat to Love* offers a complete program to discover a new way to relate to food, which requires more than knowledge; it requires a spiritual and compassionate approach to self-care."

MEGRETTE FLETCHER, MED, RDN, CDE; co-founder of The Center for Mindful Eating and co-author of *Eat What You Love, Love What You Eat with Diabetes*

"A truly delightful application of Buddhist wisdom and self-care to how we view our body image and our relationship with food. Jenna has a refreshing writing style that calls out the myths behind the diet culture that we live in and challenges the cultural norms that keep us oppressed and disempowered. A great book that guides you to tap into the empowered warrior woman in all of us."

MELAINIE ROGERS, MS, RDN, CDN, CEDRD-S; founder and CEO of BALANCE eating disorder treatment center™

"I love *Eat to Love*. It gently guides readers into a peaceful relationship with food, body, and self through understanding, attitudes, and practices that speak to the human spirit. With this book, you can shed beliefs that create real problems for health and happiness, and reawaken your innate ability to take care of yourself. Self-care never felt so good."

MARSHA HUDNALL, MS, RDN, CD; president and co-owner, Green Mountain at Fox Run; past president, The Center for Mindful Eating

"In *Eat to Love*, Hollenstein masterfully guides her readers away from the traps and empty promises of diet culture to the spiritual gifts of happiness and inner peace cultivated through meditation practice. Writing from both her personal life experiences as a 'magical eater' and her expertise in nutrition and meditation, Hollenstein empowers us all to shift our allegiance from diets to our inner wisdom, and she compassionately shows how in doing so we become more con-nected with and appreciative of our bodies. *Eat to Love* is a true gift to the world, and I am grateful to own such a valuable resource to recommend to others."

JENNIFER KREATSOULAS, PhD; author of *Body Mindful Yoga: Create a Powerful and Affirming Relationship with Your Body*

"In a sea of diet insanity, *Eat to Love* is a safe island paradise. In this deeply thoughtful book Jenna Hollenstein teaches an accessible but transformative practice for changing your relationship to your body, your eating, and yourself. As a feminist life coach, I work with women on their body image all the time, and I'm thrilled to now be able to integrate the effective mindfulness-based practices that Jenna teaches in these pages. Whether you have an established meditation practice, are new to the whole idea, or just want to find something to help you cut through the noise in your mind around food and eating, this book has what you need."

KARA LOEWENTHEIL, JD, master coach; host of the *UnF*ck Your Brain* podcast and creator of *UnF*ck Your Brain: A feminist blueprint to creating confidence*

"Jenna Hollenstein has written a beautiful, thought-provoking book about acceptance—acceptance of our bodies, of all that we are, vir-tues and flaws, and of our spiritual path. She teaches us to trust our internal wisdom, let go of 'magical eating,' with its companion belief that our bodies need to change, and helps us find our way there through a practice of patience and compassion. This valuable book is a must-read for all health practitioners."

ELYSE RESCH, MS, RDN, CEDRD, FAND; co-author of *Intuitive Eating* and *The Intuitive Eating Workbook*; author of the forthcoming *The Intuitive Eating Workbook for Teens*

"You can't practice body kindness without first connecting to your body. Mindfulness and meditation have been transformational in cul-tivating my gentle, compassionate caregiver voice. *Eat to Love* offers a deep exploration of some of my most beloved meditations uniquely delivered in the context of eating. If you would like to heal your mind, body, and food connection, this book is your next must-read."

REBECCA SCRITCHFIELD, RDN, EP-C; author of *Body Kindness*

"In *Eat to Love*, Jenna uses Buddhist teachings and principles to help guide us toward a less stressful, more satisfying experience with food. Her use of case studies and reflective questions invite the reader to examine the disconnection between the physical body and the spiritual self. This is important work for people who have spent years (even decades) in pursuit of thinness, but now crave a peaceful relationship with food and their bodies. Whatever you do, don't rush through this book. *Eat to Love* is something to be savored."

MELISSA TOLER, writer and Body Justice advocate

"*Eat to Love* is a must-read for anyone who struggles with emotional eating, food obsession, and body shame while craving peace with food, self-care, and self-love. Meditation teacher and leading authority in Intuitive Eating, Jenna Hollenstein transfers the Buddhist and scientifically supported principles of mindfulness and self-compassion into an easy-to-understand-and-follow guide that promotes readers' journeys on their Eat to Love path. Readers emerge with a rediscovery of joy inherent in eating and being in their bodies, which ultimately enhances the lives they lead."

TRACY L. TYLKA, PhD, FAED, professor of psychology, The Ohio State University; editor-in-chief of *Body Image: An International Journal of Research*

"Combining spiritual wisdom and practical strategies, Jenna dispels the myth of 'magical eating' and offers a deep understanding of how to be at peace with food and one's body. If you're ready to consider how meditation practice can help you heal your relationship with food, this book is for you! If you're already in the arena of spiritual practices—and view mindful eating to be a weight loss method—I implore you to learn from Jenna."

JUDITH MATZ, LCSW; co-author of *The Diet Survivor's Handbook* and *Beyond a Shadow of a Diet*

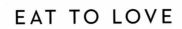

EAT TO LOVE

JENNA HOLLENSTEIN

eat
to
love

A Mindful Guide to
Transforming Your Relationship
with Food, Body, and Life

For Mom, Melissa, Lily, and Stella.
You're perfect just as you are.

ISBN 978-1-7322776-3-2 (paperback)
ISBN 978-1-7322776-4-9 (ebook)

Every reasonable effort has been made to contact
the copyright holders for work reproduced in this
book. Some names and identifying details have
been changed to protect the privacy
of individuals.

This book is not intended as a substitute for the
medical advice of physicians. The reader should
regularly consult a physician in matters relating
to his/her health and particularly with respect
to any symptoms that may require diagnosis or
medical attention.

Produced in consultation with Page Two
www.pagetwobooks.com
Cover and interior design by Taysia Louie
Printed and bound in the United States of America

eat2love.com

CONTENTS

WHAT IS EAT TO LOVE? 1

1 "YOU AREN'T GOOD ENOUGH" 13

2 A SPIRITUAL PROBLEM
   REQUIRES A SPIRITUAL REVOLUTION 47

3 THE PARAMITA OF GENEROSITY 73

4 THE PARAMITA OF DISCIPLINE 117

5 THE PARAMITA OF PATIENCE 137

6 THE PARAMITA OF EXERTION 165

7 THE PARAMITA OF MEDITATION 181

8 THE PARAMITA OF WISDOM 197

9 THE REST OF YOUR LIFE 213

   APPENDIX A: MINDFUL EATING EXERCISE 221

   APPENDIX B: TONGLEN MEDITATION 223

   APPENDIX C: LOVING-KINDNESS
   MEDITATION FOR THE BODY 227

   APPENDIX D: RESOURCES 231

   ACKNOWLEDGMENTS 235

WHAT IS EAT TO LOVE?

AT TO LOVE won't help you lose weight. You will not find suggestions for slimming down, toning up, eating clean, or being your best self. This book will not tell you how to detox, cleanse, go gluten-free, or cut out sugar or carbs.

Still reading?

Then you might want to know that, while it won't help you lose weight, Eat to Love will help you lose the destructive and unfounded belief that you will only be happy, healthy, and confident if you achieve a certain weight. It will help you drop your shame, confusion, anxiety, and paranoia about food, eating, and living in the body you have right now. It will help you shed the suffering created by the diet culture's magical eating and free your mind and body from its stranglehold.

"Eat to love" is an expression my mom used. Usually it was when recounting a dinner she cooked for someone and how they "threw their ears back and ate to love." To me, this meant eating with a sense of unselfconscious joy. It also implied an emotional connection with the food, whether it was a favorite childhood dish or something associated with cherished memories. The way my Uncle Rob ate corned beef and cabbage or my Aunt Min dove into a bowl of *spaghetti con aglio e olio.* I named my non-diet nutrition therapy practice Eat to Love with the hope that I could help women rediscover the joy inherent in eating and in being in their bodies. It was only later that I realized Eat to Love had a deeper meaning.

For many of us, eating has become fraught with worry and fear. We often eat what we think we *should* and not what we *want*. We think wanting, in and of itself, is dangerous and wrong. Or we don't know what we want anymore because, as Caroline Knapp writes in her book *Appetites,* our desires have become "submerged and rerouted." The deeper meaning of Eat to Love, therefore, is to eat as a form of self-love and care. To choose foods that give us pleasure and that feel good in our bodies. To treat ourselves overall as if we deserve happiness and pleasure just as we are.

Eat to Love also means feeling comfortable inhabiting the bodies we have right now. Everything we experience between the moment we are born and the moment we die happens in our bodies. From performing bodily functions to experiencing divine ecstasy, our bodies are there with us constantly as a vehicle and as a witness. Our bodies are intersections of race, class, gender, sexuality, and ability. They move through a world that imposes ideals and values based on these intersections, and so no body is ever the same or ever has the same experience. In our bodies, we experience pleasure and pain, strength and weakness, illness and recovery. In our bodies, we experience existential questions, deepest meaning, and spiritual awakening. Our bodies define us as separate individuals and connect us with others. Yet bodily pursuits, such as those pertaining to wellness, usually leave out our spiritual side, while spiritual pursuits, such as understanding the meaning of our lives, fail to include the body. Eat to Love recognizes that body and spirit cannot exist without each other.

This book is a call to action and a call to sanity. It brings your physical body together with your spiritual self in order to mend the separation that has alienated you from your own intelligence, pleasure, and satisfaction. It is an approach to food and body that cracks you open and connects you with what you were born knowing, as well as with the deeper values that were neglected while you counted calories, chained yourself to the scale, and watched your world, but probably not your body, get smaller and smaller. On the Eat to Love path, you are likely to find yourself thinking and being in the world differently, in part by asking how you might live your life if bodies of all different sizes, shapes, colors, ages, and levels of ability were celebrated.

Eat to Love works on two levels. The first brings a sense of attention, gentleness, and sanity to how you relate to food and your own body through the inward examination and understanding of your thoughts and feelings. The second gradually explores ways to turn that gentleness and sanity outward through the actions you take, the behaviors that define your life, and how you relate to other people, situations, and your environment. As you learn to relate to yourself and to others with kindness rather than aggression, you gradually make the world more sane and enlightened. Continually coming back to consult your heart with curiosity allows you to see beyond the narrow programming of the diet culture. The more curious you become about yourself, the more curious you become about others. The more you understand yourself, the more you understand others. And the more you love yourself, the more you love others.

By reading this book, doing the contemplations, and learning to treat yourself with gentleness, you are changing not only your own life but also the lives of those around you. Modeling compassion and attunement is a radical act in this weight-obsessed, fat-phobic, magical eating culture. Trusting your body and going beyond this insanity encourages others to take notice, perhaps planting a seed that will ripen in the future, allowing them to begin their own path. This slow outward branching increases the compassion quotient of the world we live in.

How It Works

In this book, you will learn why much of what you think you *know* about dieting, fat, and health is wrong. You will see how many of the eating and exercise thoughts and behaviors considered normal in our culture are actually harmful and disordered, marked by anxiety, obsession, and fear. I will identify for you why fat is not the problem, diets are not the solution, and our pursuit of the perfect diet or body has shoved us further away from the safety we sought toward greater pain and chaos. Finally, you will find out why seeing your body as a problem to be fixed will always lead to confusion and suffering.

Next, you will explore what it means to Eat to Love in your own life: to feed your body in a way that permits you to live (and love) your life and to connect more authentically with your world. The foundation of Eat to Love is a breath-awareness meditation practice called shamatha, also known as the practice of tranquility. Meditation, or choosing to place your attention on an object such as the breath, is inherently a process of feeling, being with, and allowing things to be as they are. In practicing meditation, we allow ourselves to be as we are. We tame our minds and open our hearts in a way that allows us to make friends with ourselves without changing ourselves. Though it might seem that the way to do this is to cast out the things we think are bad and accentuate what we consider good, that type of friendship is superficial and conditional. By practicing meditation and being with things as they are, we see ourselves honestly, without diminishing or aggrandizing anything. As a result, we develop the capacity for unconditional friendship with ourselves.

Upon the foundation of a meditation practice, Eat to Love applies a set of Buddhist teachings called the Six Paramitas, or transcendent perfections: generosity, discipline, patience, exertion, meditation, and wisdom. The Six Paramitas guide us to eat peacefully, wisely, and sustainably. If you are new to Buddhist philosophy and meditation, be assured that these concepts will be introduced in a basic sense before I address them in the context of food, body, and caring for yourself. If you have an established meditation practice and are already familiar with the Six Paramitas, know that this book will be looking at them in ways that are likely to expand your own understanding and application of them.

The Six Paramitas guide you to rely on your body's internal wisdom rather than on external forces such as diets and "experts." When you Eat to Love, you make choices primarily based on physical sensations, such as hunger, fullness, and what feels good in your body. You eat with absolute permission, pleasure, and joy. And, as a result, you are present, precise, and flexible.

Throughout the book, I offer suggested contemplations that will help you bring the power of these teachings and practices into day-to-day life. By doing them, you will develop a new language with which to describe your relationship with food and body—a language that goes beyond the narrow orthodoxy that forms bonds between dieters or clean eaters, reaching deeper to articulate previously unexplored fears, aspirations, and realizations. This new means of conveying your thoughts and experiences will help you make sense of your own journey and share it with others.

To go even deeper, download the at-home program (available at https://eat2love.com/eat-to-love-at-home-program) to transform contemplations into actions. Every day of your life for the rest of your life. During the first week of the program, you will focus on one paramita per day in order to begin a sustainable meditation practice. After that, you will have the option of continuing more intensely by focusing on each paramita for a full week. As the weeks progress, you will gradually increase your meditation practice and investigate your thoughts, beliefs, behaviors, and challenges along your personal Eat to Love path.

What to Expect

Though everyone's Eat to Love path will be unique, certain stages are more likely to occur earlier, while others come with time.

The first stage of learning to Eat to Love is recognizing how much the diet culture's magical eating promises have misled you, how dieting causes long-term weight gain, how our cultural programming makes us fear fat, and how many of us have sought security somewhere it could never be found. Part of this new insight includes how much magical eating has cost you personally. Totaling the time, money, effort, and experiences lost unsuccessfully trying to change your body is a jarring but necessary precursor to shifting your allegiance away from false idols and toward your own intelligence.

At this point, you will begin to reclaim control over how you eat and inhabit your body. Taking back this power involves removing externally or self-imposed deprivation, and eating with a sense of absolute permission, so that you discover what truly satisfies you. Appetite drives what you eat while internal sensations of physical hunger and fullness drive when and how much. By eating consistently throughout the day and nourishing your body in ways you find uniquely satisfying, you will invite and become familiar with the sensations you previously ignored or overrode.

With awareness of physical hunger comes awareness of its absence. When the desire to eat begins to arise in the absence of physical hunger, Eat to Love will guide you in choosing whether to eat or to meet your emotional needs without food, though the choice is always yours, judgment-free. By elucidating your habitual misuses of food, you will recognize patterns, reveal deeper emotions and needs, and determine how to attend to them with precision and gentleness.

Later stages on the Eat to Love path are likely to include recognizing and responding to the feeling of fullness or the sensation of *enough*, bringing joyful and embodied movement back into your life, and accepting your body as it is. Recognizing and responding to fullness is notoriously more complicated than hunger for many people. As a dieter, you subsisted on as few calories as possible, so that when you were dieting, less was more, and when you gave up on a diet, more was more. Dieting also taught you to defer to serving sizes, measuring cups, and mental tallies to dictate how much you ate rather than trusting your own physical sensation of fullness. By continuing to work with absolute permission to eat, you are allowing yourself to gradually understand what enough feels like in your body: to eat as much as you really want and need, knowing that this may change from one day to the next.

Diet culture conveyed that exercise should be a means to an end, that end being weight loss, weight maintenance, or improved fitness.

Though there is nothing wrong with exercising for health reasons, the entanglement between physical activity, weight loss, and fitness has robbed us of simple pleasures like sports, dance, and play. Moving our bodies is an inherently joyful expression of ourselves. When we bring embodied movement back into our lives, we fully inhabit our bodies and connect with ourselves and with others. Whether in how we walk, salsa, sit on our meditation cushion, or make love, it is only with the realization that our bodies are completely acceptable, lovable, and good as they are that we can delight in moving them in ways that give us the most happiness.

The penultimate stage of the Eat to Love path is accepting your body as it is right now. Acceptance could be mistaken for resignation, but nothing is further from the truth. The diet culture confused us into thinking that hating (or at least distrusting) our bodies would motivate us to change them. The truth is that such harshness beats us down and makes us feel worse, either because we drive ourselves harder or stop caring completely. Put simply, we take care of things when we love them, our bodies included. Instead of feeling as if we are surrendering the battle with our bodies to accept them as they are, we can reframe it so that we choose not to fight. Instead of waging warfare, on the Eat to Love path we aim to listen to our bodies. We vow to come back to them again and again to figure out what they are telling us. By remaining open to what our bodies are communicating, we begin the process of acceptance. Acceptance might look differently from what you expect. It does not mean never having another negative thought or feeling about your body. Rather it means committing to being with your body as it is and listening and responding to its changing needs to the best of your ability. There is no easy or quick way to do this, and this part of the process, above all others, happens at its own pace. But the rewards are deep and enduring.

You will know that you are in the final stages of Eat to Love when, more often than not, you eat without struggle, experiencing satisfaction in your food choices. When you Eat to Love, you choose foods as often for enjoyment as for how they make you feel and speak to yourself with compassion. Even though this is the final stage, this path does not end. It lasts the rest of your life, as your body continues to evolve and change.

Change is the ultimate reality. Each of us progresses through the stages of birth, growth, and puberty. Some of us menstruate, some have children, some breastfeed. Gradually we move through perimenopause and menopause. We experience countless injuries, illnesses, recoveries, and scars. From our very first moment on the Earth, change is constantly happening in our bodies, but we are often only aware of this later in life. By acknowledging the constant nature of change and committing to be with ourselves as we are, we continue to deepen our connection with our bodies, examine the nature of our minds, and stay with our true experience.

As we do this, our bodies find their natural weight, one we can sustain without struggle or deprivation and by responding precisely to internal sensations of hunger, fullness, satisfaction, and preference. You might find it difficult to imagine letting go of the attempt to strongarm your weight, but as you explore this path and all the different components of your experience, your thoughts about weight and weight loss will shift. Though this is a very active process, you do not need to *do* anything to find your natural weight. Your body will take care of it for you.

Who Eat to Love Is For

Eat to Love is for anyone who has struggled with eating and their body at any time in life. Whether you are a worried eater, a casual or chronic dieter, or someone who has faced an eating disorder, this book will help you come back to the intelligence of your own body and heart. That said, depending on your individual experience, there are different ways you can work with this material.

(A note to men: this book has been written primarily for women. Women are the principal targets of the diet culture and magical eating and have a unique relationship with food and their bodies. That is not to say that men are not affected, but since I am a woman and work primarily with women, I decided to tailor it to their experience and needs. Because the impact of the diet culture on our relationship with food and body is so primal, many of the practices here are appropriate regardless of gender.)

Eat to Love is not a substitute for appropriate and individualized medical care for anyone who has experienced an eating disorder or other mental health disorder that has affected your ability to consistently care for yourself, regardless of whether or not you have received treatment in the past. Please consider using this book as a complement to, and not a replacement for, the formal support of a treatment team that includes a physician, mental health professional, and registered dietitian. If you are currently under the care of such a team, bring Eat to Love into your work with them and investigate how a meditation practice and the Six Paramitas could help you further your own individual path to peace, sanity, and recovery. If you are not currently working with a treatment team, please explore some of the resources at the end of this book to identify someone to support you. While it may be tempting to take a self-help approach, it is particularly dangerous for those who are experiencing an eating disorder or any mental illness to be isolated while trying to drastically change their approach to eating and body image. You do not have to do this alone. The very act of asking someone for support is brave and is likely to be empowering and liberating. And I cannot emphasize this enough: If you are working with acute or chronic trauma, please consult with a medical professional immediately to determine whether meditation is appropriate for you at this time.

On the other hand, if you fall more in the gray area of unpeaceful eating—perhaps you are a casual dieter who dabbles in cleanses, couch-to-5k challenges, and thirty-day sugar detoxes, or you're a lifetime member of a certain multibillion-dollar weight-loss company—Eat to Love will reorient you to a sustainable way of caring for yourself. I actually love working with people in the gray area: those who don't meet the diagnostic criteria for an eating disorder yet are not at peace with food and their bodies. Your eating and body-image issues may not raise the reddest of red flags, but you may still be dramatically affected by these struggles and could fly under the radar for much, if not all, of your life.

Whatever unique experience you are coming from, I am so glad you are here. You have chosen a new path. It is one on which there are few right and wrong answers but where there is much respect for the wisdom you already possess. It is a path that will guide you toward a peaceful, satisfying, and joyful relationship with food and your body.

Two caveats before we jump in. First, I am deeply inspired by Buddhist teachings and cannot help but view my work through this lens. Buddhism is a tradition that encourages sincere practitioners to join its teachings with their lives, so, naturally, I have contemplated and taught classic Buddhism in relationship to food and our bodies. But these ideas are my own. Any misunderstandings are also my own and not to be attributed to any of the wonderful texts or perfect teachers mentioned. Second, as an educated, middle-class, able-bodied, thin white woman, I enjoy a significant amount of privilege as I move through the world. I have endeavored to use this privilege to offer something useful to all of us who inhabit a woman's body. That said, I am certain I have fallen short in some areas due to the nature of my experience. I am still learning and look to you as readers and fellow seekers to share with me any thoughts that would benefit this work and us all.

1

"YOU AREN'T
GOOD ENOUGH"

In the Beginning

Eating was so much simpler when we were little. First there was just one thing on the menu and it came from a breast or a bottle. Soon our options expanded and there were more tastes and textures to provide pleasure and sustenance for our adventures. We ate when we were hungry, stopped when we had enough, and knew what we liked and didn't, even if that changed by the minute. Our bodies provided endless entertainment and allowed us to explore and play. We didn't track grams, points, or exchanges, or worry about gluten or GMOs. We were blissfully unaware of the number on the scale or the little tag in our clothes. Each chunky thigh, bulging cheek, and pudgy bottom was caressed and adored. We were clear about our needs. Intuitive and satisfied.

Then something changed.

At ages as young as five, we began to look at food and our bodies differently. Maybe we overheard parents, siblings, or friends criticizing their own bodies and talking about what they should and shouldn't eat. Or we observed people being praised for their beauty and thinness, criticized for eating too much, or, worst of all, mocked for being fat. The images of women and girls in magazines and on social media, in movies and on TV (even in cartoons), and our dolls and toys revealed that how we look is the most important thing about us. Beauty and thinness were our most valued currency. Despite the changing fashion trends, thin is always in, and one false step could send us down the fearsome path of weight gain.

Suddenly the foods we ate and how our bodies looked attracted attention and became fair game for schoolyard whispers and taunts. So we internalized that criticism and that thin ideal, and we self-scrutinized preemptively. We saw our bodies as problems to be monitored, controlled, and changed. We mentally dissected our bodies into the parts we liked (those that made us likeable to others) and the parts we did not (the ones that needed to be fixed or improved to garner love and acceptance). Thoughts like *My legs are strong and help me run and play* mutated into *My legs are too chubby*. Self-criticism and harsh judgment became the new soundtrack constantly playing in our minds.

Eating became fraught with uncertainty and doubt. We questioned what we once knew to be true about our bodies. What used to be clear feelings of hunger, fullness, and pleasure were now suspect and possibly misleading. We doubted our judgment about what, when, and how much to eat, and we wondered whether our bodies could be trusted. We feared that our favorite foods were dangerous and learned to hate what made our bodies different.

Many of us tried to change our bodies by altering how we ate and exercised. We stopped listening to our internal knowing and instead turned to those outside of ourselves—fad diets, nutrition and weight-loss experts, celebrities, and well-intentioned family, friends, doctors, and dietitians—to give us the answers. Though our focus narrowed to food and our bodies, our deepest desires were for inclusion, acceptance, and love.

If your particular relationship with food and body didn't start to feel funky during childhood or your teen years, perhaps it was during a different transition. Various life events, both positive and negative, jolt us into obsessing over food and body. Divorce, infidelity, the difficulty in striking a work-life balance (particularly as a mom), a newly empty nest, a child's marriage, becoming a grandmother, caring for aging parents, death and loss, the changing work environment, perceived competition with younger women, or retirement: throughout life, women are the targets and victims of a voracious industry that creates problems with our bodies and then sells us the solution.

This is not a new phenomenon. The business and the politics of controlling women's bodies are as old as commerce itself. Every time there is progress for women, there is a commensurate backlash, usually focusing on our bodies. After the Nineteenth Amendment granted women the right to vote came the flapper age, with bound breasts, "slimming" treatments, and idealization of the lithe physique of a preadolescent boy; this was the same era in which the first Miss America contest was introduced in Atlantic City. About the same time as the second-wave feminist movement was beginning in the 1960s, Weight Watchers was born and a model known as Twiggy was heralded as the epitome of female beauty. More recently, in the 2010s, we had our first female presidential candidate in the U.S., someone who was the most qualified and prepared (male or female) to ever have run for that office. But instead we elected an inexperienced man whose claim to fame was being a reality TV star and sexual predator. You can't make this stuff up. With every political, economic, and social gain for women, the retaliation has been swift and purposeful. The message is clear: Remember your place.

No matter when we started down the destructive path of dieting and magical eating, we had no idea how far it would go or that it would reach into every aspect of our lives and cost us so much. We never predicted that funneling so much of our energy and efforts into changing our bodies to increase our confidence and happiness would, ironically, rob us of those very things. As we obsessively tracked, weighed, and measured food and our bodies and compared ourselves with impossible ideals of beauty, thinness, and perfection, we relinquished joy, fun, and pleasure. Even if we did manage to lose some pounds, with them went self-trust, any hopes and dreams not related to food and body, and our limited resources of money, time, effort, and enjoyment. When we stopped losing weight, we didn't fault the diet or the expert. We despaired over our own failure, further alienating us from our inherent wisdom.

Even though every other woman in our lives endured the same struggle—our sisters, mothers, aunts, daughters, and friends—we felt very alone. We kept it hidden and thought we were the only ones who didn't have this whole eating thing figured out. We never expressed the confusion, shame, and isolation that resulted from engaging in this losing battle with our bodies, making us even more vulnerable to the next diet that came along.

We got lost.

My Story

My dieting story began, innocently enough, at the age of thirteen, while watching Robin Wright as Buttercup in *The Princess Bride*. On the screen Buttercup is tall and slender. Her blond tresses reach to her waist and occupy as much mass as her willowy torso. When she is sad, she neither sleeps nor eats; she exists above these basic human needs and remains ethereal and effortlessly beautiful. In the final scene, she leaps from the castle window and floats down in slow motion to land almost silently into the waiting arms of the giant, Fezzik.

I remember thinking to myself, *If I jumped out of a window into someone's arms, I'd flatten him.* As the credits rolled, I looked in the mirror at my shoulder-length brown hair and wondered how long it would take until it stretched down my back. (I only now realize that she probably had extensions.) I inspected my shoulders, hips, and legs, squeezing my thighs from behind to make them appear thinner. I wished I were narrower and less muscular. In a smaller body, I imagined, I would no longer feel social anxiety; boys would desire me, girls would admire me. The route to happiness was clear: become a thinner, smaller, blonder person.

Hair color and stature aside, I focused on what I thought I could control and stopped eating. I tried not to think about my mom's good cooking and embraced the tight gnaw of hunger in my belly, envisioning how much better life would be when I transformed into someone else. This rarely lasted longer than twenty-four hours.

Of course, Robin Wright is four inches shorter than me, has a smaller frame than mine, and is a different person. And the images on which I was basing my inferiority and longing were literally a fairytale—one that clearly equated female desirability with beauty, meager appetite, and perfect breasts, but a fairytale nonetheless. In comparing myself with Buttercup, I diminished the many and varied qualities that composed who I was and focused solely on external appearance, assuming that hers was superior to mine. Suddenly, something I long suspected became a realization: my size and weight were markers, inversely proportional, as it were, to my worthiness and lovability.

I see now that this conflict was not really about my weight; it was about desiring love, inclusion, and acceptance. But I did not comprehend that at thirteen. Even after I gave up striving for Buttercup's graceful proportions, I continued to struggle with eating and my body for a long time to come.

Growing up in the late 1980s, I asserted my autonomy by eating junk food whenever not under the watchful eye of my nutrition- and weight-conscious mother. Taller than most of my friends, I felt gawky and unfeminine. I slouched to take up as little space as possible and carefully avoided walking over sidewalk grates for fear of the sound they made beneath my mass. Still, as a reluctant high school athlete, I came home after classes to comfort myself in deep bowls of hot, buttered pasta with cheese from a can (while watching *The Oprah Winfrey Show*) before returning to the freezing cold gym for basketball practice.

I endured emotionally wrenching shopping trips in which my mom and I negotiated whether to buy the size that fit or the smaller one I vowed to fit into shortly. I learned that black was slimming, horizontal stripes were not; I learned to highlight where my body was narrowest and to camouflage where it grew wide. Listening to my mom recount the weight-loss success stories of her friends, I learned that one had lost enough weight that she no longer took up the entire toilet seat when she went to the bathroom; it was then I realized that even in my most private moments I had to be vigilant about presenting my body. Returning home from my first year at college, I was at my highest weight ever, having gained steadily through the latter years of high school plus the obligatory "freshman fifteen." That summer I went on a diet (with my mom) in which I drastically lost weight by subsisting on industrially produced, tasteless low-fat meals, listening to inspirational weight-loss cassettes while sweating on a plastic lounge chair in the backyard, and satisfying my craving for peanut butter by inhaling a deep whiff as I sailed through the kitchen. (I loved my mom's howls of laughter at that last part and how close I felt to her even though I couldn't wait for that diet to be over.)

Returning to college as a sophomore (and choosing my major in nutrition), I was armed with new knowledge of how to fill up on vegetables, forgo midnight pizza gatherings, and assuage cravings with artificial sweeteners and processed diet foods. As I continued to lose weight through completely disordered behaviors, the new attention I received made it clear that weight loss was worth any cost. Later, as a first-year nutrition graduate student at Tufts University, I was lonely, depressed, and at my most unbalanced, eating-wise. I drank too much cheap red wine from a jug and compensated for those calories by surviving on steamed vegetables and stool softeners. Meanwhile, my best friend referred to me as "fit and flare" because of my penchant for outdated-yet-flattering dresses that highlighted my waist and hid my hips.

Throughout my dieting career, I tried the grapefruit diet, the cabbage soup diet, the master cleanse, low-fat diets, low-carb diets, SlimFast, Jenny Craig, Weight Watchers, Atkins, South Beach, juice cleanses, eating cleanses, and good old-fashioned restriction. I learned not to drink my calories, to box up half my restaurant meal the moment it was served, to opt for the lighter version of anything good, to weigh and measure my food and myself, and not to trust my body. What I did not know during this time, and what was largely unknown to many dietitians and the medical community, is that diets are not sustainable for a variety of biological and emotional reasons and, in fact, do much harm.

Magical Eating and the Diet Culture

In a parable made famous by David Foster Wallace (that likely dates back to Confucius), two young fish are swimming along when they happen to meet an older fish swimming in the opposite direction. The older fish nods at them and says, "Morning, boys. How's the water?" The two young fish swim on for a bit until eventually one of them looks over at the other and says, "What the hell is water?"

Water, for the purposes of this book, and to understand the origins of our food, eating, and body thoughts and behaviors, is the diet culture we all swim in. It's the one that tells us we'll be happier, healthier, and more lovable if we just lose the weight or find the right diet. The culture in which, 99 percent of the time, beauty is depicted as young, white, thin, cis, and heterosexual. The culture of fashion labels that refuse the potential multibillion-dollar revenue stream from millions of willing women who live in average-size or above-average-size bodies so as not to dilute their brand. The culture of constant surveillance of women's bodies in Hollywood for being too fat or too thin, for gaining too much while pregnant (*She better be careful!*), for gaining too little while pregnant (*How vain!*), for losing the baby weight too fast or too slow, for having cosmetic surgery, for not having cosmetic surgery, for dressing too old, for dressing too young. The culture that monitors every pound lost or gained by Oprah, Jessica Simpson, Kirstie Alley, Britney Spears, Kim Kardashian, and Kelly Clarkson. The culture that pathologizes food restriction, over-exercise, and obsession in too-thin bodies but encourages and congratulates it in fat bodies. The culture of insidious and ubiquitous fat shaming, even in children's books and cartoons. The culture of *The Biggest Loser*, *My 600-lb Life*, *Celebrity Fit Club*, *My Diet Is Better Than Yours*, *Shedding for the Wedding*, and *Extreme Makeover*. The culture of shockumentaries like *Supersize Me*; *Food, Inc.*; *Forks Over Knives*; *Fed Up*; *What the Health*; *Food Matters*; *Hungry for Change*; and *Fat, Sick and Nearly Dead*. The food-obsessed culture of *Top Chef*, *Iron Chef*, *Chopped*, *Chopped Junior*, *American Diner Revival*, *Baconation*, *Beat Bobby Flay*, *Cake Hunters*, *Cake Wars*, *Cupcake Wars*, *Carnival Eats*, and literally hundreds more. The culture that publishes endless headlines about the obesity epidemic, complete with decapitated images of fat bodies, yet never misses a chance to highlight the supposed health benefits of drinking wine or eating chocolate. The culture that publishes studies that fail to prove higher weights cause chronic health problems yet conclude that it is "still wise to achieve and maintain a healthy weight." The culture that established bariatric surgery as the gold-standard solution for the "problem" of unruly, fat bodies even though it carries risk of death, surgical complications, repeat surgeries, malnutrition, micronutrient deficiency, alcoholism, depression, and suicide. The culture that proclaims this dangerous procedure an ultimate solution by completely disregarding the human beings on the other end of the knife. And the culture in which it is acceptable to discriminate against people of size, denying them the same access to jobs, healthcare, education, and other social benefits because being fat is supposedly their choice.

Like those young fish, we are entirely immersed in the diet culture and unable to avoid its endless current of images from traditional and social media, stealthy marketing and advertising campaigns, and the world of biased healthcare professionals who force-feed us weight-loss guidance hidden in mistaken warnings about ill health. Because we swim in these messages for so long and from such an early age, we come to see them as truth. And because we are assured that we can change our bodies if we only try hard enough, we become trapped in a cycle in which we deprive our bodies of energy and satisfaction for the end result of weight loss. Finally, dieting becomes unsustainable because we stop losing weight, rebel against the deprivation, or both, and the pendulum swings violently in the other direction, leading us to binge on the very foods we forbade ourselves and to forsake any health-promoting behaviors we did while dieting, causing us to regain any weight lost and often then some.

Swimming in the diet culture gives rise to what I call "magical eating": the search for the diet that will lead to peace, endless happiness, and an end to our suffering. Magical eating comes in many varieties. The Weight Watcher keeps returning to the same system that "worked" for her in the past, even though her weight has gradually crept up with each stint. The Revolving Door Dieter has tried everything and is up for anything; she has down the basics of "eat less, move more" but is searching for the next gimmick that will help her solve her weight "problem" for good. The Health Food Junkie is all about organic, non-GMO, and avoiding adrenal fatigue and can be found spending 50 percent of her paycheck at the health food store (unless you catch her on an off day, when she has a box of Entenmann's devil's food crumb donuts for dinner). The Boot Camp Devotee takes everything to a higher level; her workouts rival basic training regimens and her diet is all about shredding muscle and obliterating fat. The Accidental Vegan controls her body primarily by having fewer options on her menu and masks her food anxiety with eating righteously. The Lifestyle Changer had a come-to-Jesus moment with a physician, whether over a fasting blood glucose result or knee pain, and vows to do whatever is necessary to defend a healthier (i.e., lower) weight for the rest of her life. The Fearful Eater may be found hovering over a menu or in a grocery store aisle, fretting over which foods cause weight gain, inflammation, and embarrassing gastrointestinal distress.

Whatever its particular variant, magical eating creates the most convincing advocates of the diet culture in us. As we internalize its overt and covert messages, we reinforce the diet culture in how we talk to and treat ourselves and others. We become free promotional labor for the diet industry, promoting its interests inwardly and outwardly so that it is nearly impossible to opt out. And with our undeniably strong purchasing power as women, we support the very products and services that further oppress us. As a result, we end up spending more on beauty and body-related products than on education. Sadly, because of our magical eating, we are more likely to suffer from depression, anxiety, disordered eating (and, in some cases, eating disorders), and to have lower self-confidence, ambition, cognitive function, and achievement. This is a direct result of the message that our worth is based on our weight and of that message's impact on our thoughts, feelings, behaviors, and how we live our lives.

Magical eating and the internalization of the diet culture's value system creates a soundtrack that plays nonstop in our minds, sometimes loud, sometimes barely perceptible, but always there, sculpting our self-image and driving our choices. It narrows our focus so that all we think about is what we should be eating, how to resist eating what we want, how to burn the most calories for our effort, and how to fix what is wrong with our bodies. That such thoughts occupy a disproportionate amount of our mental real estate alone makes magical eating unacceptable and unsustainable, but the impact of this dysfunctional relationship with food and our bodies goes beyond our daily lives, and indeed beyond our own bodies.

In more far-reaching ways, magical eating affects what we strive for in life, what we prioritize, and how we contribute to the world. It alters how we educate ourselves, what professions we choose, who we befriend, how we partner, and how we think we deserve to be treated by others. It defines whether we spend time, effort, and money on diets and cosmetic procedures or on things aligned with deeper, more meaningful values. It determines whether we surround ourselves with people equally obsessed with weight and appearance or with those who expand our minds and challenge us to grow. It dictates whether we ask ourselves what gives us joy and whether we pursue those goals or if we delay our happiness until we feel we deserve it.

In the 2011 documentary *Miss Representation*, Katie Couric asserts, "If women spent a tenth of the time thinking about how to solve the world's problems as they think about their weight... we could solve them in a matter of months." The dissonance between our magical eating and our true values has an impact on how women's interests are represented locally and globally, how we continue to be objectified, and how we are disproportionately affected by violence. Though women make up 51 percent of the population, we comprise only 20 percent of Congress. We are not just victims here; we are also the perpetrators, voting to uphold this imbalance. Until we recognize how we contribute to our own oppression, whether in the political system or in the diet culture, the greatest opposition to women's progress will continue to be other women.

As Lindy West writes in her heartbreaking memoir *Shrill*, "When you raise every woman to believe that we are insignificant, that we are broken, that we are sick, that the only cure is starvation and restraint and smallness; when you pit women against one another, keep us shackled by shame and hunger, obsessing over our flaws rather than our power and potential; when you leverage all of that to sap our money and our time—that moves the rudder of the world. It steers humanity toward conservatism and walls and the narrow interests of men, and it keeps us adrift in waters where women's safety and humanity are secondary to men's pleasure and convenience."

Diets Don't Work

Much of what we consider common sense about diets is false. Body weight cannot be simplified to calories in/calories out, eat less/move more, and you just have to try harder. Dieting often leads to a pattern of weight-loss-and-regain, also known as weight cycling, which is actually associated with many of the negative health consequences usually attributed to being in a bigger body in the first place. What's more, research is showing that, of the fairly limited things we have some control over, it is behavior that is a better predictor of overall wellness across the spectrum of body shapes and sizes. To illustrate, consider this scenario.

CHERYL IS 5 foot 7 and has, in her own words, "always struggled with my weight." In high school, she weighed between 150 and 155 pounds, which was bigger than most of her petite friends. So Cheryl was continually on a diet, coming off a diet, or thinking about going back on a diet. With each diet, she initially lost some weight but eventually regained the pounds, often with the addition of a couple more. Whenever she was not following a specific diet, Cheryl had a tendency to overeat the foods she thought of as fattening or bad for her. Now, at thirty-five, Cheryl works as a VP of a large healthcare marketing firm. She was just asked to be the maid of honor in her best friend's wedding, taking place in eight months.

It's Monday morning and Cheryl steps on the scale: 184 pounds. She resolves to eat no more than 1,200 calories per day and to work out five times per week until she reaches her goal weight of 150 for the wedding. She feels motivated, in control, and excited about how she'll feel when she's lost the weight. For breakfast, Cheryl has two hard-boiled eggs, an apple, and black coffee. When mid-morning hunger hits, she ignores it, thinking she can last until lunch, which consists of a salad with grilled chicken and dressing on the side, no bread, and a bottle of artificially sweetened fruit-flavored water. She works through the afternoon, responding to the gnawing feeling that strikes at 3 p.m. with another cup of black coffee. She declines after-work drinks and goes straight to the gym, where she burns 600 calories on the elliptical (according to the machine's computer). Coming home, starving, Cheryl pops a frozen low-carb burrito in the microwave and anxiously stares as it rotates, illuminated, on the little glass tray. She burns her fingers removing it from the package and devours it standing over the sink, half noticing that it was chicken when she meant to grab the beef. Pleased with her restraint, Cheryl brushes her teeth and collapses into bed early to prevent herself from eating any more, which is fine because she's exhausted anyway.

Tuesday and Wednesday look similar, except for an "incident" with the cookie tray during Wednesday's afternoon meeting. For a few hours afterward, Cheryl berates herself but resolves to undo the damage with an extra half-hour on the elliptical. She is heartened to see the scale edge down to 182 pounds and regards that as proof that her diet is working.

By Thursday morning, Cheryl feels less motivated and more sluggish. She is about to run out of eggs and is not sure when she will have time to pick up more. She trudges through her workday in a fog and wonders if she might be coming down with something. She phones in her workout, cutting it short by twenty minutes, and wearily slinks home, snacking on whatever she finds in her cabinets because she lacks the energy to even put anything in the microwave.

On Friday morning, Cheryl oversleeps, grabs a breakfast sandwich on her way into the office, and skips lunch to balance out her indiscretion. She snaps at a co-worker when asked for her thoughts on a shared account. At an after-work gathering, margaritas are accompanied by nachos, which Cheryl digs into heartily though she barely tastes them. She vows that they will count as her dinner. Back at home, still tipsy, she orders takeout delivery of a cheeseburger, fries, and chocolate milkshake and eats them mindlessly while binge-watching Netflix, easily bypassing the point of comfortable fullness. She awakens on the couch the next morning surrounded by evidence of her binge and decides to toss her new diet out the window for the next two days.

Saturday and Sunday consist of unrestrained eating, especially of foods she resisted all week: ice cream, pizza, and her favorite, macaroni and cheese. Cheryl doesn't make it to the gym that weekend (actually, she doesn't even leave her apartment). She cancels plans with her friends and isolates herself, feeling terrible. She finishes up all of the forbidden foods in the house on Sunday with the plan to start over Monday morning, when she steps on the scale again: 186.

In this oversimplified but familiar scenario, Cheryl starts off feeling in control and excited about losing weight. She easily follows prescriptive dieting rules such as minimizing the calories she takes in and maximizing the calories she burns. Her eating choices are driven by what she believes will lead to weight loss rather than by what appeals to her, and she ignores natural hunger and fullness sensations when they arise. She takes an all-or-nothing approach by throwing in the towel (on a program that was unsustainable anyway) when she slips up. And she reacts to her perceived failure by overeating foods she believes are forbidden, not even allowing herself to enjoy them.

This illustrates just a few of the serious physical and emotional repercussions of restricting to lose weight. Our bodies need energy from food regularly throughout the day in order to function. None of us gets around this. Not eating enough makes us feel tired, irritable, and depressed. It stresses our bodies and immune systems and may lead to changes in mood, poor sleep quality, and illness. When we eat fewer calories and nutrients than our bodies need, strong compensatory mechanisms kick in to help our bodies fight what they perceive as starvation. We get exceptionally hungry and food actually starts to look and smell more appealing. We become preoccupied with food and eating and can think of little else. The instinctive drive to eat when restricted may lead us to crave different foods than we are typically hungry for, such as those that are high in sugar. We may also eat too fast, bypassing the gradually emerging sensations of fullness and eating to an uncomfortable point of fullness, missing out on true enjoyment and satisfaction.

Restriction is the best predictor of increased intake of the restricted food. Case in point: our current dread of sugar and carbohydrates has led many to restrict their intake of these foods, only to find themselves binging on the very same foods. While many think this is proof that sugar and carbs are addictive, the scientific evidence does not support this. The primary flaw of studies that claim to prove sugar addiction is that they do not take into account the effects of restriction; without excluding individuals who restrict high-sugar foods (or even think that they should) there is no way to prove that sugar is addictive. There are famous studies that position two functional MRI images of the brain side by side: one on heroin, for example, and one on sugar. They claim that because the pleasure centers of the brain light up in both images, both substances act on the brain similarly. What they do not include is how the brain lights up while walking outside on the first beautiful spring day, falling in love, or having an orgasm. One of the cornerstones of addiction is a drive to acquire the desired substance in any form. This is why you cannot have mouthwash when you check into alcohol rehab. But if I placed a bowl of sugar in front of someone who believed they were addicted to sugar, would they dig in? Would you?

Not eating the foods we want creates a growing feeling of deprivation that elicits rebellion even in the most mild-mannered of people. Restricting ourselves in this way conflicts with our natural drive to assert our autonomy; it inevitably backfires when we can think of nothing else but what we are *not* supposed to eat. This may result in aggressively eating *at* someone or something—at our non-compliant bodies, the burden of restriction, the feeling of deprivation, the patriarchy—in a way that also doesn't correspond with our actual physical sensations. The physical and emotional effects of restriction not only make it nearly impossible to stay on a diet, they also trap us in the binge-restrict cycle. And diets change the way we relate to our bodies in terms of movement. By making exercise obligatory for the purposes of weight loss or control, we lose the connection with our bodies and any joy derived from being in them.

Had Cheryl maintained her diet for more than a week, here's what likely would have happened. She would have continued to lose weight for a short time. When she reached about 5 percent weight loss, or 175 pounds, a series of biological changes would set in. Her body would become more efficient, effectively learning to subsist on fewer calories, causing her weight loss to plateau. Not seeing further loss, Cheryl would choose to (A) continue her diet but feel frustrated and confused at not continuing to lose weight, (B) restrict even more, compounding her body's compensatory mechanisms and eventually plateauing anyway, or (C) quit her diet and resume her previous eating pattern.

The body's ability to adapt to less energy coming in is an evolutionary benefit, and the ability to become more efficient by storing fat should be credited with the survival of the human race. Historically, when people experienced famine or just inadequate food sources, they didn't die. Good news for them. But barring situations of true scarcity (which absolutely do happen more than we realize and seriously complicate things for a person living with limited access to a variety of foods in this diet culture), many of us in today's land of plenty only face a perceived famine when we impose it on ourselves. (One might see the minimization of body fat as an expression of our current privilege, compared with the privilege of eras past in which bigger bodies were considered desirable and preferred—but I digress.) And because the body adapts to fewer calories, resuming the higher-calorie diet on which we maintained a higher weight may actually cause us to gain more weight—meaning that if Cheryl had chosen path C, she would have likely been in for a rude awakening.

This is how we diet ourselves up in weight by increasing our set point range, as depicted in the image below.

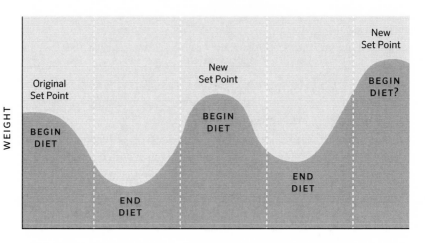

This phenomenon was the subject of a 2016 research article in the journal *Obesity*, which studied contestants from the reality TV show *The Biggest Loser*. What they found was that the contestants' weight loss slowed their metabolism more than would be expected, given the actual changes in their bodies. Even years later, contestants' bodies had adapted to the diets they had been placed on to such a degree that they needed fewer calories than would be predicted to sustain their body weights, even though most of them had gained back significant weight.

What used to be known as yo-yo dieting scientists now refer to as weight cycling, and they have found that it actually has more negative health effects than can be directly linked to being in a larger body in the first place. Physically, the negative health effects of weight cycling include increased overall illness and heart disease. Emotionally, weight cycling is associated with increased distress, greater risk of binge eating and eating disorders, lesser likelihood of being physically active, lower self-esteem, and greater idealization of thinness. Not exactly what they highlight on those late-night diet system ads. How ironic is it that these are the actual outcomes of a process we initially engaged in to alleviate our suffering?

In Cheryl's scenario, her goal was to weigh what she had in high school, when she first started to diet. Each of us has a natural weight or set point range that is determined by several things that are simply out of our hands: genetics are the strongest determinant; economics and geography affect access to preventive health care, places to be physically active, and nutritious foods; and the family food environment in which we are raised provides us with norms in terms of beliefs, habits, and practices that are positive or negative for eating and body image. Many people who have been dieting for much of their lives look back at photos of their younger selves, at times they remember being so uncomfortable in their bodies and wanting desperately to lose weight, and wonder, *What was I thinking? I was so cute!* Or, as one of my clients put it, "Now I wish I was as fat as the first time I thought I was fat."

Considering all the genetic, physiologic, emotional, and economic barriers to long-term weight loss through dieting, there is clearly something wrong with our assumption that success is simply a question of willpower. Think of this: if Weight Watchers worked, they would put themselves out of business. Instead, they are casting a wider net to target teenagers to meet their revenue goal of $20 billion by 2020. Companies like Weight Watchers thrive because of a repeat business model in which dieters keep coming back again and again. When we do lose a few pounds, we credit the diet, and the diet creator is happy to accept this credit. When diets don't work, which is about 90 percent of the time, we blame ourselves, and the diet creators are quick to point out our shortcomings (and offer us half off our next purchase). Failing to lose weight through dieting makes us turn on ourselves, seeing ourselves as failures and our bodies as untrustworthy. And as we shift our attention to finding a new diet, we act out Einstein's definition of insanity: doing the same thing over and over again and expecting a different result.

Fat Is Not the Problem, Fat Stigma Is

Much of the diet culture and our magical eating are based in a fear of becoming fat. This leads to a stigma, bias, and even phobia toward fat. But before touching on fat stigma or weight bias, I would like to talk about the word "fat."

For many of us, the word fat is loaded with implicit negativity. But please grant me a chance to argue that the word is actually a more sane, honest, and unbiased option than currently acceptable terms like curvy, full-figured, overweight, or obese. Curvy and full-figured emphasize what we begrudgingly consider positive aspects of being in a bigger body, such as having sexually alluring curves or full features such as breasts and hips. Overweight and obese, on the other hand, are medical terms that indicate there is a standard normal weight that you can be either above or far above. The word fat, absent the malicious intentions with which it is often used, is neither positive nor negative. It is not inherently an insult just as thin isn't inherently a compliment. It is just a word used to describe a bigger body or a body with more adipose tissue than the currently accepted norm. As counterculture as it may be, we have a choice to reclaim the word fat if our bodies have more adipose tissue, recognizing that this neutral descriptor is still laden with meaning for many others. Even reclaiming this word and confidently inhabiting your bigger body is a form of activism. The Fat Acceptance Movement, also known as Fat Liberation and Size Acceptance, which began in the late 1960s, was closely tied to the feminist movement and has similarly occurred in waves.

Why do most of us consider it common sense to think that being fat is unhealthy and wrong and being thin is healthy and right?

Dieting to lose weight, get fit, and improve health is not just condoned in our society, it is heartily encouraged by much of the medical community. After families, doctors are the strongest advocates of fat bias. But authors Linda Bacon and Lucy Aphramor outlined in a 2011 *Nutrition Journal* article and in their 2014 book *Body Respect* how many of the medically rationalized messages with which we have all been inculcated are false.

1. Fatness does not decrease lifespan. Studies show that people categorized as overweight have longer lifespans than normal-weight people and those categorized as mildly or moderately obese live at least as long as normal-weight people.
2. Fat's role in poor health is exaggerated. While certain diseases are found to occur more commonly in bigger bodies, that does not mean that disease is *caused* by fat. The increase can be explained by fitness levels, weight cycling, and, as I will show later, discrimination.
3. The body mass index is not a useful measure of one's health. The BMI is a relatively arbitrary ratio of weight to height created by epidemiologists to study populations, not to classify individual bodies.
4. Scientific evidence does not show that exercise and dieting are effective methods to lose weight long-term (as I already discussed, with Cheryl as my example).
5. It has not been proven that weight loss improves health. Studies have shown that behaviors such as exercise and eating nutritious foods improve wellness, but this is regardless of a change in weight.
6. Finally, the biggest contributors to our health, which include genetics, economics, and access to healthcare, are not under our control.

I know these points may be difficult to swallow. But what is important to grasp here is that much of what we hold true about weight and health was based on poor-quality scientific evidence that has been and continues to be debunked. Since the misinformed genie has gotten out of the bottle, however, it has been virtually impossible to put him back in. And as someone who has read the studies and observed personally and professionally the damage that dieting does, it sometimes seems that no amount of scientific data showing that fat is not the problem and diets do not work will dissuade even the most educated of medical minds from believing just that.

Pathologizing fatness has contaminated the judgment of many medical professionals to the extent that we cannot always rely on them to properly and objectively guide us on the care and feeding of our bodies. This is important to acknowledge because it highlights the fact that all of us—scientists, doctors, and dietitians included—have our biases. And in many cases, a bias against fat and people in bigger bodies affects our ability to deliver impartial and appropriate care to all people. Couple this with being a member of any marginalized group—women, non-white, disabled, gay, trans, or non-binary—and fat stigma is amplified.

I have also observed (unscientifically) that the fat stigma possessed by the formerly fat—those who *were* able to lose weight and keep it off by making it their full-time job—can be quite invective. While it is true that some people lose weight and keep it off, it is statistically very rare, and we simply do not understand all of the factors that have made this possible for a few but not for most. And when it does happen, the extreme efforts of exercise and dietary restraint required calls into question whether it should be considered successful and healthful, or disordered. However, the common "if I could do it, anyone can" perspective that results has served to sell many a diet book and spread shame and fat bias.

Because our culture prizes thinness, this is the lens through which we exist, relate to one another, and perpetuate ideas and ideals. The trickle-down effect is that many of us have internalized this notion and are projecting it onto ourselves and others, even if it is not based in accurate scientific evidence and even if it causes us much physical and emotional harm. Because of the media's blanketing of every visual channel with ultra-slim photoshopped models and our internalization of thin ideals as unequivocally desirable, we have developed a collective cultural bias against fat. This socially acceptable prejudice, with its many parallels to sexism, racism, and homophobia, has instilled the belief that not only are fat people unattractive and unsavory, their weight is also a matter of choice, completely under their control. For people in bigger bodies, this means a lower chance of getting a job, of being treated fairly and respectfully, and of being accurately seen (and objectively diagnosed) as a whole person by medical professionals.

In a 2014 *Journal of Obesity* article on an approach to health that prioritizes wellness over weight, Dr. Tracy Tylka and her co-writers define weight stigma (also known as fat stigma or fat bias) as "negative weight-related attitudes and beliefs that manifest as stereotypes, rejection, prejudice, and discrimination toward individuals of higher weights," and link it to feelings of body shame, body dissatisfaction, eating disorders in women, and disordered eating in men. Fat stigma may, in and of itself, drive unhealthy behaviors due to learned helplessness; if people in bigger bodies feel they are automatically viewed as unhealthy, they may not do the healthy things that they enjoy and that feel good, including engaging in preventive medical care, eating nutritious foods, exercising, and caring for their mental health. Another study found that watching the TV show *The Biggest Loser* increased fat stigma, decreased motivation to exercise, and solidified negative stereotypes of fat people. This is why *how* we think about weight affects our weight. If we saw weight as one more individual characteristic, largely out of our control, much like hair color, we might discover the unique ways in which we enjoy eating and moving our bodies. And we might be more inclined to take care of our bodies simply because they are precious and deserve such care.

A different approach recognizes that a variety of body shapes and sizes can be compatible with health and wellness, and that weight loss via dieting has a multitude of unintended negative consequences on health. When the shame and learned helplessness of bias against fat is taken out of the equation, people are free to connect with internal determinants of what, when, and how much to eat; what types of movement their bodies prefer; and what other behaviors they wish to engage in for the purpose of wellness. Put simply, when free from fat stigma, it is possible for all bodies to achieve health and wellbeing.

Yet diets remain monolithically prominent in mainstream culture. With about half the American population trying to lose weight right now (that's almost 180 million people) and spending major coin to that end ($66 billion in 2017, according to a Marketdata research report), one might conclude that dieting has replaced baseball as the national pastime. Why?

Diets are seductive. They make empty but attractive promises. Even though we may have been at our current weight range for most of our lives, diets promise to make our dreams of being smaller come true in just a few days. We all know what seems too good to be true usually is, and diets are no exception. Diet advertisements predictably make unrealistic claims about the effectiveness of their product, highlighting enviable success stories with dramatic before-and-after images, yet include this statement in microscopic print at the bottom of the TV, computer screen, or magazine page: *Results not typical.* Part of us knows we are being lied to, or at least manipulated, but we want so badly to believe that we overlook the shady parts. The resulting cognitive dissonance between what we know from our own lived experience of magical eating and what we want to be true only compounds our confusion.

Diets have also shape-shifted over the years. Recently, as wellness and mindfulness have become popular, certain words and phrases coined by the non-diet and body-positivity movements have been co-opted by people and companies still selling weight loss. By doing this, they make their product or service sound like it is not a diet. But let me assure you in no uncertain terms: if someone or something is telling you what, when, or how much to eat or exercise, no matter how much they tout self-love, it is a diet.

The best predictor of the future is the past. Yet despite all the personal and scientific evidence that diets don't work, we can't seem to help but hope for new ways to lose weight. Though scientists continue to come up empty in their search for proof of food or sugar addiction, dieting itself becomes an addiction, with all the associated highs and lows. You take someone in whom nothing is wrong, distort body image by suggesting only the thinnest bodies are desirable and worthy of love, and introduce the idea that their own body should not be trusted so that they get trapped in the binge-restrict cycle. Then they think they need diets to solve the problem that diets created in the first place. One subset of the Fat Acceptance Movement, a feminist group known as The Fat Underground, coined the wonderful saying: "A diet is a cure that doesn't work for a disease that doesn't exist."

Often when we experience something positive, pleasurable, or ecstatic, the pleasure center in our brain lights up. The seduction and anticipation associated with dieting, particularly at the beginning, as well as the feelings of virtue and belonging that a diet brings us, all give us great pleasure. Why else would we keep coming back? Our optimistic brains (and every piece of marketing or advertising we consume) tell us that what will finally fix our problematic bodies and make us happy at long last might be just around the corner. And so we keep looking. Even scientists and physicians think like this. Rather than deciphering how to be well in the bodies we have (a wellness-over-weight approach that is based on good evidence), they continue to search for better ways to lose weight, even opting for dangerous solutions such as bariatric surgery in increasing numbers.

Finally, we should never underestimate the power of magical eating as evidence of the systemic oppression of women. Because it is framed as being good for you, good for the economy, good for the healthcare system, and good for others, dieting essentially becomes a social obligation, one that is mainly targeted at women. When you're told that you're worth nothing unless you're thin, what choice do you really have? This is how dieting becomes a form of survival. If you're in a fat body, you must become thin. If you are in a thin body, you must not become fat. No matter what size or shape our body, we are affected by this oppression, which we, in turn, consciously or unconsciously perpetuate. This deepens our phobia of fatness, which furthers fat stigma, and on and on.

Your Magical Eating Won't Save You

Eating is an inherently sacred activity; we take something from out-side of our bodies and make it part of ourselves. It is both universal and very personal. But more and more our eating practices and the particular foods we embrace or eschew seem to have greater mean-ing for us. They represent how we view ourselves and our bodies on a larger scale, how we believe our choices will affect us now and in the future, and even what is inherently right and wrong. The sacred nature of eating could be celebrated by making choices based on a connection with our bodies or compromised by letting forces outside ourselves drive our decisions.

In what I call my blissfully ignorant phase—the period of my life before I started my first diet—it had not yet occurred to me that any-thing was wrong with my body. At some point, I remember hearing my mom lament her own weight, worrying that her good cooking (she was known around the neighborhood for the dishes she left at people's doorsteps when they had a death in the family) conflicted somehow with her children's ability to stay thin. At dinner one night, Mom said, "We could all stand to lose a little weight."

"Please pass the potatoes... wait, what?"

Growing up, I received mixed messages: I was loved for who I was, but being thin and beautiful would make me even better. I would have better assured safety, acceptance, and inclusion, things that I (and the rest of the human race) deeply craved. Instead of eating accord-ing to hunger, fullness, and satisfaction, I felt a greater emphasis on eating what I could get away with as long as it didn't cause weight gain and substituting diet-compliant foods for what I really wanted. This had the obvious effect of grouping foods into the categories of *good* and *bad*; foods that were less enjoyable were more likely to lead to thinness and foods that were desirable would supposedly make me fat. Though I heard whispers about eating disorders in my extended family, what was still implicit was the suggestion that we could always be thinner, more beautiful, a little better. It was only with a lot of time, therapy, and perspective that I saw the flaws in the seductive but dangerous idea of "never enough."

The subtle aggression of never enough stops us from ever relaxing with ourselves as we are. We might delay doing what we love, postpone new experiences, or defer treating the bodies we have now with respect. Instead of living our lives fully and appreciating the present moment, we channel all our attention, energy, and hope into an uncertain future in which we might become worthy of love and acceptance from others and then, perhaps, from ourselves. The belief in never enough lurks at the heart of much of our magical eating, and it is exquisitely malignant because it suggests we could always lose one more pound, tone those thighs or upper arms just a little more, or make our diets even more clean and pristine. These aspirations are not without serious repercussions.

How the media portrays thin people conveys subtle and not-so-subtle messages about youth, beauty, and desirability, and how they relate to power, control, and health. If we were thin and/or found the perfect diet, we would suffer less, live better lives, and be happier. We are also told that weight is completely within our control, that being thin is possible for everyone, and that if you are not thin, it is because you are not trying hard enough. Here lies the nexus in which dieting ventures into the realm of a spiritual practice.

When you think of spirituality, you might evoke a set of rules that show you the way to inner peace, to ending your suffering (and possibly even avoiding death), and to being good. On the darker side, it also evokes the fearful consequences of not following the rules, an inability to question them, belief in myth, and possibly even a fear of pleasure. (Remember the frozen yogurt episode of *Seinfeld*? "How could this not have any fat? It's too good!")

Throughout the ages, people have attempted to make sense of the world through spirituality and religion. Besides offering guidance on how to live a good life and how to treat one another, many religions have food-related laws and traditional practices. Catholics eschew meat on Fridays during Lent, Jews who keep kosher never eat pork or shellfish or mix meat with dairy, and Muslims observe the holy month of Ramadan in part by fasting between sunrise and sunset. What and when food is eaten or not eaten is often part of how people identify themselves, demonstrate belief, and practice their faith.

As the number of Americans formally identifying with a particular religion continues to drop, those who identify with a diet or manner of eating has risen dramatically. But there are many similarities between religious eating practices and the fervor that surrounds many diets today: they are driven by belief, imbued with morality, and carry a sense of identity and community. Even the language we use to describe food and eating smacks of religion. We avoid what is *sinful* or *taboo*, we feel *guilt* for giving into *temptation*. *Miraculous* weight-loss tricks pique our interest. We practice *rituals* of food procurement and preparation in our pursuit of dietary *purity*. We *cleanse* and *eat clean* to rid the body of *impurities*. Even the words *good* and *bad*, when applied to food, are a strong interpretation of the adage "you are what you eat."

The pursuit of thinness through dieting can be likened to our previous search for a connection with the divine in that it provides a sense of purpose and meaning. Diets present a philosophy to believe in and a moral code to observe. They organize our days, weeks, months, and years with rituals that provide safety and structure. Most importantly, diets provide instant community, a feeling of belonging, and connection with others.

Being thin can be framed as being near godly, and it is often the underlying motivation even when dieters claim their eating choices are driven by health instead of weight. In fact the number of people who admit to following a specific diet has decreased in recent years, likely representing more people "eating for health" rather than for weight loss. Spoiler alert: lifestyle change = still a diet.

Take the Paleo diet, in which people consume only those foods eaten by our Paleolithic ancestors between 2.5 million and 10,000 years ago. Proponents claim that this is how our bodies were designed to eat before the dawn of agriculture, industry, and modern diseases such as obesity, heart disease, type 2 diabetes, and cancer. The Paleo diet consists primarily of foods that could be hunted or foraged, such as meats, fish, nuts, seeds, berries, roots, and tubers. It shuns dairy, grains, lentils, beans, peas, peanuts, and other legumes that were not in existence during this period of dietary correctness.

Public proponents of this diet, which takes some doing, say they have never felt better and that it cures everything from acne to arthritis. But those statements are invariably overshadowed by the diet's emphasis on weight loss. Online Paleo forums provide a platform to share before-and-after photos of shrinking bellies and abdominal, arm, and leg muscles gradually becoming more defined. Meanwhile, followers forever seek ways to recreate their favorite starchy foods: zucchini noodles; spaghetti squash instead of spaghetti (my Sicilian partner would die); brownies made with nut flour, coconut oil, and agave; and endless manipulations of cauliflower to simulate rice, mashed potatoes, pizza crust, the bread on a grilled cheese, and even ice cream.

I don't mean to pick on the Paleo diet. It does convince people (at least those who don't binge-eat in reaction to its restrictions) to eat fewer processed and more nutrient-rich whole foods. But it misses the mark on many levels. By avoiding foods that are the result of agriculture and industry, Paleo dieters neglect many nutrients, including dairy sources of calcium, whole grain sources of fiber and minerals, and bean and lentil sources of protein. The claim that Paleo dieters simulate the diet of their ancestors is not just false, it is impossible; the diet is at best a rough approximation of what our cave-dwelling ancestors ate, because as we have evolved, so too has the nutrient composition of the diet's permitted plant and animal foods. And claims of improved health through the Paleo diet are somewhat misrepresented; studies show that even during their short and treacherous lives, our Paleolithic ancestors had cholesterol in their arteries, and today's much longer lifespan (that continues to lengthen) suggests not everything that has developed during the last 10,000 years has been to our detriment.

Other ideological diets are also often rationalized by scientific-sounding claims not representative of the full body of evidence, unintentionally misinterpreted, intentionally misrepresented to sell something, oversimplified, or exaggerated. But perhaps the most compelling aspect of these types of popular diets, ones that have supposedly revolutionized people's lives, is their subtle promises of safety and salvation. Without saying it outright, they intimate this idea: *By eating these sanctioned foods, you will suffer less, avoid disease, and enjoy the eternal peace and happiness that naturally come from being thin, healthy, right, and good.*

If all this is not enough to convince you, magical eating—which includes all of these different attempts to control the way we eat in order to make sense of chaos—provides a sense of structure, belonging, and identity. The moral superiority dieters acquire from eating righteously often leads them to proselytize, sharing how their diet has cured all that ailed them, given them renewed energy and purpose, and provided lasting peace.

Our religious fervor for magical eating hints at something larger than a preoccupation with body fat percentage. Like religions of the past, magical eating has become our modern-day attempt to make sense of a confusing, uncertain, and chaotic world. We all want to live good, happy lives of meaning and purpose. But how do we do that? How do we know if we are doing it right? With whom do we compare ourselves? How is progress measured?

The black-and-white thinking espoused by magical eating and the blind faith it requires provide a clear definition of success. We weigh and measure our food and our bodies to determine if we are on the right track. By following the rules, we are assured we are constantly improving, living virtuously, and moving in the right direction. We feel we are regaining control amidst the chaos and confusion, and living with a degree of certainty and security.

Unfortunately, it is a false sense of security. We cannot truly control our environment or avoid suffering, and the world will continue to be an uncertain place. Our attempts to control the uncontrollable through magical eating quickly fail or take over our lives as in the case of eating disorders, disordered eating, the binge-restrict cycle of chronic dieting and weight cycling, or any of its various incarnations. As a result, we are left even more confused, uncertain, and out of control than when we began.

BROOKE DESCRIBED HERSELF as a "chubby" kid. Her family joked that she ate butter with a spoon directly from the butter dish while sitting in her highchair. After a horrible breakup in high school, Brooke developed gastrointestinal problems consisting of alternating diarrhea and constipation. Between her GI problems and not knowing their cause, Brooke and her family became very worried and anxious, which led Brooke to develop panic attacks. Her loss of appetite led her to suddenly and unintentionally lose a significant amount of weight, and she began to receive new attention from her peers. By the time Brooke was diagnosed with "likely irritable bowel syndrome," she had made the connection between being thinner and feeling safe and accepted. Brooke adopted a nearly fat-free diet to master her body. Fast-forward twenty years and Brooke was raising two children and working as an advertising executive for a women's fashion company. When she came to work with me, she shared how her unpeaceful eating had come and gone over the years but was particularly triggered with the birth of her son, which was approximately the same time her daughter was diagnosed with a rare pediatric cancer. Though her daughter was now in remission, Brooke's eating and exercise regimen had become more rigid and now dictated her life. Her fixation shifted from the dangers of fat to the perils of sugar and she became very active in a gym that specialized in high-intensity-interval training (HIIT). Her husband felt she was always at the gym and thought it ironic that she was so fixated on perfecting her body when he barely saw it anymore and they rarely had sex. During meals, Brooke ate different foods from what the rest of her family did, and this was not lost on her kids. Her daughter started to show signs of restrictive eating and several times expressed that she was afraid of becoming fat. Though she was resistant at first, wishing only to focus on food, Brooke eventually conceded to working with a therapist skilled in anxiety and eating disorders. As the three of us partnered over the course of more than a year, Brooke connected the dots between her strong emotions and her eating and exercise dysfunction. As she gradually allowed herself to fully feel her scariest emotions—fear of losing her child, anger at not having control, sadness at the loss of time and presence with her family as she maintained strict adherence to her diet—she found she could loosen her grip on eating and her body, allowing herself to have more flexibility, show up more, and embrace her beautiful imperfections.

Our desire to make sense of the world represents good intentions, but attempting to do so by manipulating our bodies backfires. If we follow the route of dieting to feel happier; to connect with others physically, intimately, and emotionally; or to feel confident in ourselves and in our lives, it only takes us further away from those very things. It is the worst example of the carrot and the stick, in which being fully engaged, demonstrating our love for others, feeling joy and confidence in our bodies and in our world are all experiences we continually postpone until the day when we are somehow different.

Instead of freeing us to engage fully with the world, magical eating imprisons us. Instead of allowing us to turn toward our loved ones and our communities, it isolates us and turns our attention inward. Instead of making our lives better, happier, and more fulfilling, magical eating makes them progressively smaller and emptier.

I am certain you have plenty of original ideas, but the one about your body being flawed and in need of fixing is not one of them. That thought was programmed into you by the patriarchal commercialism of the diet culture, by the people around you (those you trusted, admired, emulated, looked to for guidance, and those who were similarly programmed), and ultimately by yourself as you internalized the body-as-problem ideology. Yet, there is no reason for regret. Because you are seeing this clearly and with open eyes after years of delusion, and that means it is possible now to move forward with presence, honesty, and gentleness.

Lindy West closes *Shrill* with statements about "world-building activities." She describes how giving up her body hatred, the desire to please others, and a focus on the narrow landscape of changing her body instead of the larger panorama of the world's needs are all contributing to a better world. This is why we are here. This is our invitation and our potential. Authentically showing up for your children, your partner, your community, and, most importantly, yourself: this is how we make the world better. "We're all building our world, right now, in real time," she writes. "Let's build it better."

2

A SPIRITUAL PROBLEM REQUIRES A SPIRITUAL REVOLUTION

CHANGING OUR DIET or the size and shape of our bodies will never give us the spiritual outcomes of happiness and peace. That only comes from working with our hearts and minds. The greatest paradox inherent in magical eating is how we spend a disproportionate amount of our limited resources trying to remodel our physical bodies, which can only be changed so much due to our genetic makeup, the long-term effects of dieting, and many other factors beyond our control. On the other hand, we spend little time working with our minds, including how we perceive our relationship with food, eating, and our bodies, even though the mind is much more susceptible to our influence. The fact is, working with our minds is a more effective and fruitful use of our emotional (and physical) capital.

In the time before you thought there was anything wrong with your body, when you weren't afraid to eat, you valued kindness and compassion over six-pack abs or a low-carb diet. Though we cannot recreate the past, we can reconnect with the basic intelligence of our bodies in how to care for them and once again enjoy self-trust and pleasure. We possess the capacity to perceive things differently, to give less credence to thoughts that denigrate us and more to those that make us feel worthy. We do this by becoming familiar with ourselves as we are, by cultivating nonjudgmental curiosity, and willingly noticing what arises. When we give ourselves this time and attention, we begin to remember our own insight. This path unfolds over time as we choose it again and again for the rest of our lives. And the strongest support for this evolution is the practice of meditation.

My own path began about a year after I quit drinking at the age of thirty-three. Since my teens, I drank to manipulate how I felt about myself, along with my fears about how others perceived me. When I felt socially awkward, drinking eased my anxiety. When I grappled with fear, anger, loneliness, or heartbreak, it lessened my pain, if only temporarily. When I hated who I was, drinking gave me a mask to wear. Getting drunk is easy to confuse with having fun, even if it has destructive consequences. But regardless of its presentation, there is always something suspect about not being able to experience discomfort.

As I entered my thirties, I wondered if drinking was detracting from my life rather than enhancing it. Behind the lighthearted persona I tried to project, I knew I was self-medicating. By pretending to be less heavy-hearted, sensitive, and emotional, someone I thought others wanted me to be, I lived inauthentically. My drinking didn't change me into that alter ego; it brought out the worst in me. When I drank, I hurt people's feelings and was not present at all. Though for a time I believed drinking made me more interesting, it didn't do that either. Instead, it kept me small and scared, because it originated with the belief that there was something fundamentally wrong with me. What I learned in sobriety, and as I started to meditate and study Buddhism, was that all of my awkwardness, anxiety, and strong emotions were okay; they were not in need of remodeling. I didn't have to change my feelings or myself to be a happier or more lovable person. What I needed to change was how I related to difficulty. In fact, that has made all the difference. Because I had been a dietitian for so many years, I started to see the overlap between how and why I used alcohol and diets: to change how I felt, to change who I was, to be perceived favorably by others, to comply with society's standards of happiness.

Underlying our confusion about what to eat and our anxiety about our bodies is something disconcerting. We live with a perpetual sense of inadequacy, a belief that we are not okay as we are, that we are problems to be fixed. Whether or not we are conscious of this feeling of fundamental defect, we are driven to rid ourselves of this deep sense of *dis-ease*. Since we cannot identify its exact source, we identify more tangible problems: we don't live in the right city, didn't choose the right partner, don't have enough money, the right job, the right house. These problems feel less existential and more concrete; we might imagine our discomfort could be resolved by moving, renovating, changing jobs, or breaking up. Alternatively we might fixate on what is not quite right about our bodies, how they are too big or too small in certain places, not fit or toned enough, too different from the cultural ideal or from the body we had at seventeen. We make our bodies into projects, by perseverating on what's wrong and what should be improved. Monitoring the number on the scale or tracking grams of carbs gives us something solid to focus on. We think, *If I could just get that number on the scale down to X, my grams of carbs down to X, my diet a little cleaner, my life would be better, easier, I wouldn't suffer so much.* And the industries selling magical eating support this notion by providing an endless lineup of systems, tools, and programs, thereby fueling the hope that the solution is just around the corner, you just haven't found it yet, gone far enough, tried hard enough.

Thinking we need more willpower, to cut out gluten, or to cleanse ourselves to within an inch of our lives represents a fundamental misinterpretation of our predicament. Sculpting our bodies or remodeling our diets will never give us the deep sense of spiritual satisfaction we think it will. However far we take it, there will always be more to do. If, on the other hand, we were able to work with our minds and hearts—in how we perceive our experience, and in how we think, make choices, and take actions that align with deeply held values in this chaotic and constantly changing world—we might finally come to view ourselves as fundamentally fine... just as we are. The bottom line: the answer to our dissatisfaction with ourselves is not about changing our bodies but about transforming how we see them. It is not about never having negative thoughts and feelings but about relating to them differently. This forms the basis of a spiritual path.

A spiritual path is an ongoing exploration that involves paying attention to the present moment, the very ground under our feet. The word spirituality might provoke a strong reaction. Some think it has to do with religion while others associate it with new-age self-help. What I mean by spirituality is actually neither of those. It does not require conversion or asceticism, and it peacefully coexists with any religious belief you already have, even if that is a complete absence of religious belief. Spirituality is how you work with your thoughts and emotions, how you hold your mind and heart, how you live your life, and how you relate to yourself, others, and your surroundings.

The Buddha himself sought an answer to his own deep feelings of dis-ease. Born Siddhartha Gautama, the man who became the Buddha was a prince in India. He was sheltered by his father from all the causes of suffering. Even though he was surrounded only by beauty and pleasure, he became curious about what went on beyond the palace walls and insisted on seeing for himself. When exposed to the realities of suffering, sickness, and death, he was deeply distressed but felt compelled to seek equanimity amid this reality. He saw a tranquil monk and decided to leave all his pleasures and worldly possessions behind to pursue *enlightenment*, the ability to see the nature of reality and be at peace. At first he immersed himself in asceticism, severe self-discipline, and renunciation of all forms of indulgence but nearly died of starvation. He realized that self-imposed aggression and deprivation was not the path to enlightenment, and when he was well enough, he sat down beneath a bodhi tree and meditated, simply *being with* his thoughts and feelings, until he understood the nature of reality.

Part of that reality is that there are three fundamental aspects to life, which the Buddha called the three marks of existence. These are (1) the truth of suffering, meaning that suffering is a natural and unavoidable part of all of our lives; (2) impermanence, how nothing is stable or solid and everything is always changing; and (3) egolessness, or how everything is connected and there is no true separation between "me" and "you."

In *Buddha's Brain: The Practical Neuroscience of Happiness, Love & Wisdom*, neuropsychologist and meditation teacher Rick Hanson explains how these basic and inevitable parts of life perfectly align with our brain's natural survival strategies. These include the preference for pleasure over pain, the desire to make constant that which is always changing, and the tendency to "put things in boxes" to better understand them. This means that the exact things our brains are wired to do to survive and make us feel safe, the things we think will make us happy, are actually the things that cause us pain. This might sound like cause to give up, but I see it as reason to relax. Once we see that it is natural and normal to resist the three marks of existence, we can finally begin to work toward relaxing with them: to acknowledge that suffering is inevitable and expand to accommodate it, to recognize impermanence and develop gratitude for the present moment without getting attached, and to see how we are all connected, and so develop compassion for others struggling with the same reality.

The Buddha discovered that constant amusement, protection, and royalty did not give him perfect, lasting happiness, and neither did cutting out all pleasures and living with the bare minimum. Indeed both extremes were aggressive means of resisting the three marks of existence. Instead the Buddha sought to find a balance, or *a middle way*, in which he could be with the full spectrum of human experience and maintain equilibrium and steadfastness. Not to master or control his life but to ride the experience as it continued to change. This is our goal as well: to observe the millions of variations between extremes, understand what drives us to such polarities, and work toward discovering our own middle way.

The teachings of the Buddha, known as the *dharma*, help us discover the middle way by emphasizing working with our own minds, where our suffering originates, and learning how to apply the resulting insight in our everyday lives. The dharma connects us with core values by creating space around deep-seated beliefs and helping us to develop new ways of looking at them. For these and many other reasons, the dharma is relevant to our relationship with food and our bodies.

In addition to being known as the teachings of the Buddha, the word dharma also means *the path* and *the truth*. Unlike some religions (and forms of magical eating) that require blind faith, the dharma is meant to be considered, questioned, and tested. Nothing should be taken to be the truth until you have tried it out in your own life and observed the results for yourself. The way to do this is through the practice of meditation. In simply sitting and being with your thoughts and feelings as they are, you too possess the potential to discover the nature of reality.

The reason a meditation practice is so critical to seeing things as they are is because it changes the structure and function of the brain. Meditation increases gray matter in the regions of the brain called the anterior cingulate cortex, which controls self-regulation, attention, and cognitive flexibility; the prefrontal cortex, which governs executive function, planning, problem solving, and emotional regulation; and the hippocampus, the part of the limbic system that affects learning and memory and that is very sensitive to stress. Meditation also decreases brain cell volume in the amygdala, the part of the brain that controls our fight-or-flight response, and weakens its connection with the prefrontal cortex, which translates to less reactivity. Functionally, the frontal lobe, or the most highly evolved part of the brain, quiets down; the sensory processing of the parietal lobe slows down; the thalamus slows the influx of sensory inputs; and a part of the brain known as the reticular formation decreases arousal. As a result, the brain sharpens, becoming less reactive and more skillfully responsive. The changes we encounter as the result of our meditation practice are not limited to our time on the cushion; they extend into every part of our lives when we practice with consistency.

It is worth noting that our practice is done with open eyes. This cultivates an additional layer of stability and open-heartedness because we never retreat inward; instead we remain steadfast amidst our everyday environment. Sitting with open eyes is inherently a practice of wakefulness that supports the development of a peaceful relationship with food and our bodies.

The Buddha saw things as they are through the practice of meditation. Similarly, as you embark on your own Eat to Love path, your primary tool in working with things as they are is the practice of meditation. Though I examine meditation in greater detail in chapter 7, I offer some basic meditation instruction here for several reasons: so that you understand the definition of meditation as I mean it throughout the book; so that you may begin to practice the technique; and so you grasp that this is the ground upon which all the other teachings are built.

Shamatha Meditation Instruction

There are three aspects to shamatha meditation: mindfulness of body, mindfulness of breath, and mindfulness of mind.

In *mindfulness of body*, you take a comfortable seat, one that emphasizes the dignity inherent in stopping in the middle of this crazy world to work with your mind. The meditation posture is simultaneously relaxed and uplifted. If you are seated on a cushion on the floor, cross your legs loosely in front of you. If you are in a chair, sit so that your feet are flat on the floor.

Whether seated on a cushion or in a chair (both of which are equally spiritual, by the way), feel your body connect with the seat beneath you and give your weight over to it completely. Allow yourself to take up and fully occupy that space rather than trying to make yourself smaller in any way. Building from the ground up, allow your hips, spine, shoulders, and head to stack vertically. The pelvis should rest in a neutral position, neither pitched forward nor slumped backward. The spine is straight and strong with its natural curves, the back of the neck is elongated, and the crown of the head reaches gently up to the sky. The front body is open, soft, and receptive. You may allow your belly to relax and stop clenching it or holding it in, and allow the chest and heart to soften. Let your shoulders relax down your back and let the upper arms be parallel with the torso. Rest your hands, palms down, on the tops of your thighs. Play with the position of your hands so that they are neither pushing nor pulling your upper body. Try dropping your hands down by your sides, bending at the elbows, and resting your hands wherever they land on your thighs. Let the hands relax.

Release the muscles of the face and the throat. The mouth is closed, with the jaw relaxed, lips and teeth slightly parted, and the tip of your tongue resting where the back of the teeth meet the roof of the mouth. Keep your breath natural and normal, in and out through the nose; no special technique is needed. Keep your eyes open, because this is a practice of wakefulness and being with whatever arises in your real life. The gaze is soft and cast down slightly at a point about six feet in front of you. Your eyes take in the full visual field without focusing on any one spot; you might experiment with imagining that your eyes are relaxing back in their sockets or that you are looking at a point in the middle distance.

In *mindfulness of breath*, bring your attention to the physical and sensual qualities of the breath: the feeling of air on the outside of the nostrils or brushing the back of the throat, the rise and fall of your chest or belly, or the feeling of your clothing moving against your skin. How each inhale happens without your needing to manage it, how at some imperceptible point the inhale turns into the exhale, and how there is a small pause at the end of the exhale before your body breathes in again, naturally. Rather than thinking about or observing your breath, you are feeling yourself breathing: breathing in each unique inhale and breathing out each unique exhale, in the present moment.

In *mindfulness of mind*, you place your mind's attention on the feeling of the breath as if riding waves. Maintain this awareness on the breath even as you notice thoughts flickering like fireflies or passing by like clouds. Just as the eyes continue to see and the ears continue to hear, the mind continues to make thoughts. This is not a problem or something you need to stop. There is no need to "clear the mind" while you meditate; instead, you are practicing allowing your mind to be as it is, while you choose to feel the breath. If you don't get attached to them, most thoughts come and go on their own. You might envision your thoughts as being in the background of your awareness while you feel your breath in the foreground.

When you notice you have become absorbed in a line of thought, to the point that you have lost the feeling of the breath, know that this is also not a problem. Simply acknowledge the thought—you might say silently to yourself, *thinking*—and then let it go with a sense of precision, gently coming back to the feeling of the breath. That moment of noticing you have become distracted is no reason to berate yourself or tell yourself you are a bad meditator; it is actually something to celebrate because in that moment you are fully awake and have chosen to once again place your body and mind in the same place at the same time by coming back to the feeling of the breath. Noticing ourselves thinking *is* the practice, so it doesn't matter how many times your attention strays; whenever you notice that this has happened, just gently escort your attention back to feeling the breath as the object of your meditation.

The Buddha discovered the nature of reality and became enlightened by sitting down and meditating. This very same technique. Simple, but not easy. You will have questions about the breath, about the posture, and certainly about the eyes being open. These are all fine and manageable. No one is perfect at this. That is why we call it a practice. I will have much more to say on meditation in chapter 7.

Three cycles of teachings have traditionally been attributed to the Buddha. These are referred to as the three turnings of the wheel of dharma. Each turning of the wheel refers to a yana, or vehicle: the Hinayana, or foundational vehicle; the Mahayana, or greater vehicle; and the Vajrayana, or indestructible vehicle. All three levels of understanding and practice are relevant to creating a new relationship with food and our bodies, and the basis for all three cycles is the practice of meditation.

On the Hinayana path, we tame the mind by addressing the fundamental qualities of our lives: observing the basic precepts of citizenry, such as not stealing, killing, lying, or abusing intoxicants; behaving in an ethical way; and simplifying and not living in excess. We clean up our spiritual house, so to speak.

On the Mahayana path, we train the mind to move beyond our solitary experience and relate to the world in which we live. This includes other beings, our culture, and our environment. The Mahayana path is associated with softening and opening the heart.

On the Vajrayana path, which is practiced when the mind is more deeply trained in meditation and dharma, each moment of our lives presents the opportunity for enlightenment. Every thought, feeling, experience, and interaction presents the opportunity to awaken to things as they are and to see the true nature of reality. The Vajrayana path is connected to the sense perceptions of sight, hearing, smell, taste, and touch.

Philosophically, one might assume that a book about eating and body would be Hinayana because of its narrower focus that pertains to one's personal experience. But the Eat to Love approach is much vaster and deeper than this. What has become the traditional way of relating to food and our bodies through magical eating and self-aggression is too limited a way of being in the world. It ignores our basic drive to live vibrantly and to relate to one another. In learning to Eat to Love, we practice on the Hinayana path by meeting our body's basic needs. Then we expand beyond the diet culture, beyond magical eating, and indeed beyond ourselves (though we don't leave ourselves behind). We practice on the Mahayana path by cultivating compassion for ourselves and others. Because our compliance with and participation in the diet culture is self-perpetuating, opting out has a ripple effect that affects ourselves, other people, and the culture. And because every feeling, thought, and action around eating and our bodies presents us with a choice to either repeat habitual patterns or to be released from that claustrophobic view, we are also practicing on the Vajrayana path.

The Six Paramitas

Building on the foundation of a meditation practice, the Six Paramitas are a Buddhist framework that helps us make sense of the confusion and chaos inherent in our lives while also caring for our bodies in ways that are gentle, sane, and aligned with our true values. The Six Paramitas are a central teaching of the Mahayana, from the second turning of the wheel of dharma.

The Six Paramitas are: generosity, discipline, patience, exertion, meditation, and wisdom. In the following six chapters, we will delve deeply into each one. You will find that there is a natural progression from generosity to discipline, from discipline to patience, and so on. In fact, each paramita stabilizes or balances the preceding one: discipline stabilizes the practice of generosity, patience stabilizes discipline, and so on. Because the Eat to Love path is one you will travel for the rest of your life, your understanding and practice of the paramitas will continue to evolve beyond the first reading of this book. Sometimes you might come back and work more intensely with the paramita of patience, for example, or bring greater exertion to your path. As you continue to practice being with your experience as it is, the resulting insights will guide you to engage with the paramitas as needed to address your specific challenges, shifts, and changes in the way you relate to food and your body over the course of your life.

Bodhisattvas, or those who apply the Six Paramitas, make compassion their primary practice. We often think about compassion as something we have for others. But as with anything, before we extend compassion to others, we must first find it for ourselves. Treating ourselves with compassion is particularly difficult when it comes to eating and body, as most of us were taught to be harsh, critical, and self-aggressive. For this reason, we treat ourselves as we would a beloved *other*, such as a dear friend, child, or pet. Even though we are essentially our own most significant other, there are ways in which we are hidden from and unknown even to ourselves. Practicing compassion toward ourselves through the Six Paramitas is a way of taking off our own mask and getting to know ourselves with unfiltered honesty and friendliness. Because of what we have learned from the diet culture, this may seem counterintuitive, but this is a process of getting to know the real you and offering that person compassion and kindness. Continuing down this path, it will become clearer exactly how treating ourselves with compassion has the effect of spreading compassion outward toward others. As we step out of the cocoon of magical eating, we soften toward people in our lives, see how they also struggle to feel love and acceptance, and witness one another beyond the superficial confines of the diet culture. As we assume this different perspective, changing how we relate to eating and our bodies has implications for how we create positive change.

The word paramita translates as *crossing over* or *going to the other shore*. The shore we leave behind is one of suffering, while the one we are crossing over to is one of courage, compassion, kindness, equanimity, and open-heartedness. It is not that we leave our suffering behind, avoid it, or get rid of it. Rather, we bring it across with us as we learn to relate to it differently. We aren't getting rid of negative thoughts, we are changing how we relate to them; we aren't changing our body, we are changing how we relate to it. Practicing the Six Paramitas permits us to go beyond the limited, dualistic thinking of magical eating that teaches us that there is a right and a wrong way to eat, that thin bodies are the only good bodies, and that we should gear our limited resources of time, energy, and money toward changing ourselves, even if that costs us enjoyment, satisfaction, and even physical and mental health. As we cross to the other shore, we focus less on arriving and more on the journey itself. On the way, we learn to rely less on certainty and groundedness, both of which are illusory, after all, and instead we train in staying with our experience despite uncertainty and impermanence. This ability to stay with our true experience increases our flexibility and resilience in a variety of situations and states of mind.

In addition to being known as bodhisattvas, people who train in opening their hearts with compassion are also described as warriors. Not warriors who are violent or aggressive, but, as American Buddhist nun Pema Chödrön describes them, warriors of non-aggression: people who willingly venture into difficult or challenging situations to create change and help others (including themselves). Emotional first responders, if you will. Choosing the path of warriorship involves the willingness to challenge one's own sources of oppression, including fixed ideas about how we should look/eat/be that actually cause more suffering under the guise of safety, freedom, and happiness. The ultimate task of the warrior is not to figure out a way to avoid suffering, uncertainty, and fear but to learn how to relate to these forms of discomfort more genuinely. Though there is no guarantee that the warrior will find comfort, these practices provide support and stability through good times and bad.

Considering the mass cult–like programming we have endured in the diet culture, the analogy of the warrior makes perfect sense. For our own wellbeing, we must be warriors who do not accept the status quo that oppresses us and damages not only our bodies but also our confidence and self-trust. For the wellbeing of others, we must be warriors to prove there is another way of existing that is beyond the small-mindedness of magical eating.

Lojong Slogans

Up to this point, I have shown how we became alienated from our intelligence and our own bodies. You have begun to understand that the path to enlightenment, or the ability to see the nature of reality, is not in changing who and how we are but in relating to reality differently, guided by gentleness and compassion. The lojong slogans support this transformation by reminding us of basic truths we might have lost sight of or taken for granted. The coupling of the paramitas and the lojong slogans take us from an intellectual understanding to practicing new thoughts and behaviors in real time.

The slogans are fifty-nine short sayings that reconnect us with our basic emotional intelligence by cutting through distractions and distortions to reveal what we already know. The word lojong translates to *training the mind,* so these sayings are also known as the mind-training slogans of Atisha. Atisha was an eleventh-century Indian meditation master who established the most enduring lineage of Tibetan Buddhism. Though he lived a monastic life, his primary emphasis and work was on how the practice of meditation and the study of the dharma allowed all of us to be of benefit to others. The lojong slogans were created as a support for practice and study and as a means of transforming obstacles or difficulties into the path of enlightenment. They integrate perfectly with the Six Paramitas and, though we won't be looking at all fifty-nine slogans, over the course of this book I will present a selected few that can complement your practices of generosity, discipline, patience, exertion, meditation, and wisdom.

Upon first glance, the lojong slogans seem simplistic, but with continued contemplation, you might discover that they are quite nuanced, reminding you how to awaken your mind and open your heart on the spot in a range of settings, both easy and difficult, pleasurable and painful, comfortable and uncomfortable. As we continue this practice, how we relate to ourselves and to others softens, becomes deeper and more compassionate.

Now we begin. Here, I present the first lojong slogan, which comprises four reminders and provides the basis on which we build our Eat to Love practice. It helps us generate direction, motivation, and even urgency to remember what truly matters.

First train in the preliminaries

The preliminaries described in this slogan ("the four reminders") are:

1. To maintain an awareness of the preciousness of a human birth
2. To be aware of impermanence: the life of every living being ends
3. To recognize the cycle of karma: whatever you do has a result
4. To remember the unsatisfactory nature of suffering

The first preliminary, to maintain an awareness of the preciousness of a human birth, asks that we recognize how fortunate we are to have been born into a human body. When you consider all the different organisms on the Earth, it is remarkable that we were born human. We are privileged to have the most sophisticated brain of any organism (at least on this planet and as far as we know), an exquisitely crafted body that adapts to changing circumstances and virtually runs on its own (lucky for us), and a capacity to experience the world sensually through sight, hearing, smell, touch, and taste.

Having a human body allows us to do what we enjoy, to care for others, and to work with our minds so that we lead dynamic, vibrant, and meaningful lives. Even the ability to click a button and have this book delivered wirelessly is a pretty amazing thing that should not be taken for granted.

Cats can't do that. Yet. That we know of.

Maintaining an awareness of the preciousness of a human birth is also to recognize the pains and drudgery in having a human body. A body is inherently uncomfortable. From minor irritants to catastrophic injuries and disease, at times living our lives in a human body feels very difficult. Think about how narrow our window of comfort is as human beings; we only tolerate a couple of degrees change in body temperature without serious consequences. We are completely derailed, or at least seriously distracted, by irritations such as a stuffy nose, headache, or sore back. We brace against and complain about changing ambient temperatures on sweaty summer afternoons or bitter winter walks to work. We endure countless injuries, illnesses, and physical limitations. We suffer extremes of thirst, hunger, exhaustion, not being able to poop, or really needing to pee. To put it simply: having a human body is hard.

The discomfort inherent in inhabiting a human body often leads us to lay blame. Whether major or minor, instead of considering that unpleasantness might be a normal part of having a human body, we quickly fault ourselves for not doing what we could to prevent it, bemoan the need to feel such unsatisfactoriness, and immediately shift into problem-solving mode. The moment we experience some form of physical discomfort, we try to fix it by changing what we eat. Our headaches must be caused by sugar. Our acne by dairy. Our gastrointestinal distress by gluten. Our stress and fatigue must be caused by carbohydrates or some rare mineral deficiency.

Our physical dis-ease may be caused by what we are or are not eating, but the swiftness with which we blame our bodies and resort to changing our diets is worth noting. It often prevents us from taking a compassionate and common sense approach to working with the normal difficulties of having a human body. We could consider a more likely explanation for our headaches, for example, such as not drinking enough water, or that our fatigue is the result of inadequate sleep. In medical training, they teach students, "When you hear hoofbeats, think of horses, not zebras." Similarly, we might consider the most likely explanations for our discomforts rather than immediately seeking to avoid them through changing what we eat.

Also inherent in having a human body is the need to care for it. Air, food, water, shelter, warmth, and sleep form the basis of Abraham Maslow's hierarchy of needs. As I will explore in greater detail in the following chapter, we need to eat meals and snacks consistently throughout the day in order to fuel our bodies. We need to drink enough water to allow our bodies to carry nutrients to our cells and function optimally. Our bodies need adequate and high-quality rest every day in order to be able to do what they do day after day. Yet, despite these universal truths, I can't tell you how many people avoid drinking enough water so that they don't have to do the bothersome task of going to the bathroom, who don't interrupt their work momentum long enough to feed themselves, or who don't give themselves time to heal when they inevitably get sick. I've heard people lament the fact that there is not a pill that would make eating obsolete. And it is no secret that many consider how little sleep they get to be a badge of honor, as if we should be able to overcome this basic need.

Beyond our physical needs, our bodies require safety and love in order to function best. We need to feel we are included, understood, and seen by others in our immediate and extended circles. But many do not have this basic form of wellbeing for various reasons: we don't consider ourselves worthy, or we are treated as unworthy because of our race, gender identity, sexual orientation, ability, body size, or age; we are taught to fear that something sinister might be lurking in the food supply, causing inflammation, cancer, autism, and fatness; and we feel that eating is a dangerous exercise, like walking on a high wire without a net, and that one false step could spell disaster.

In maintaining an awareness of the preciousness of a human birth, we connect with our basic goodness, also called Buddhanature. In the Buddhist view, all beings possess basic goodness, which is a pure, wholesome quality that is primordial and everlasting. This is the opposite of the concept of original sin, in which we are born bad and must suffer in order to reap our ultimate reward. Basic goodness holds that we do not need to overcome anything to be considered worthy (and that suffering is a natural part of life). Joy and pleasure do not need to be earned. We begin with goodness and carry it with us throughout our lives.

Because all beings possess basic goodness, this logically extends to the bodies we live in. If our bodies are basically good, then all aspects of our bodies are basically good. In addition to the things that we like, or at least tolerate, so too are the things that we struggle to accept and the parts we never think about at all. Our ear, nose, and arm hair. Our bumps, bruises, scars, rolls, stretch marks, and cellulite. Our sniffles, colds, and coughs. Our aches and pains. All are basically good. We could also consider the basic goodness of the parts of our bodies we usually take for granted. Our immune, nervous, and circulatory systems. Our hearts pumping blood, lungs oxygenating our cells, kidneys and livers cleansing and ridding the body of waste, eyes seeing, tongues tasting, and brains processing millions of inputs every second.

When we see our bodies from the vantage point of basic goodness, we begin to take a bigger view and appreciate their miraculous entirety. How they adapt to the constant changes that occur throughout various states of growth, wellness, and illness. How we grow from a single cell into a baby, child, teenager, and then adult. How that very same body has the capacity to gestate and nourish a baby. How our bodies continue to function even when we do not take very good care of them, and how they combat germs by launching an immune response. How they ensure our survival by storing fat and do the physical work that is required for us to live our lives, sometimes resulting in aches and pains. Even if our own unique body isn't perfect in some way, if we are missing a limb, require dialysis, or don't fit the culture's narrow standard of beauty, recognizing how our bodies *do* work for us helps to remind us of the wonders that they are. Acknowledging our bodies in this way helps us move beyond the limited view of our bodies as objects to be changed, sculpted, and perfected. Instead we begin to understand that our basically good human bodies are instruments that let us live our lives and be of benefit to others.

How do you feel when you contemplate the preciousness of your human birth and the basic goodness of your body?

The second preliminary is to be aware of impermanence. The life of every living being ends. We are born, we thrive, we get old, and we die. And in between those milestones, our bodies are never stagnant; we progress through different stages of growth; sustain injuries, then recover; become ill, then recover. We feel physical pain, which, if we pay attention, waxes and wanes and also changes by the minute. Perhaps we become pregnant, grow babies, and give birth. We breastfeed or use our physical bodies in other ways to care for children and others. The bodies we had when we went on our first diet aren't the same bodies we have now; nearly every cell has been replaced. Even if nothing seems to be changing right now, our bodies are simply getting older moment by moment. Eventually all of us will die.

On the Eat to Love path, we work with our minds so that we recognize and respond to the constant changes of the body. We acknowledge and accept impermanence, cultivate gratitude for things as they are, and refrain from becoming too attached to anything. We feel our bodies grow hungry one moment, begin eating, become satisfied, and digest the food we have eaten to nourish, grow, and heal. We remain steadfast as each thought and feeling follows the predictable course of arising, leveling off, and eventually dissolving. We feel whatever natural emotional responses we have to impermanence, like sadness, remorse, and anger, and do not get stuck in aggressively resisting its inevitability.

We acknowledge that our time on Earth is precious and limited. We must choose what to prioritize in order to live according to what is most important. And we must choose what to renounce. I often think about how I will look back on my life at the moment of my death. Would I rather have spent ages chiseling and remodeling my body even into my elder years, or to have lived my life, devoured the chocolate, enjoyed the sex, and inhaled the roses? Would I prefer to have respected the culture's standards of female compliance, or to have disrupted that nonsense and challenged harmful norms? Would I rather I didn't ruffle any feathers, or feel that I had been of benefit to others, had cared for them (and myself) to the best of my ability, and had loved with my whole heart? When put that way, there's no contest.

Just as we train in meditation practice to place our attention on the breath and hold it there, we decide where to place our attention and exert our energy. We don't have to participate in a system that oppresses us, makes us miserable, and offers little in return. We have a choice of what to eliminate from our lives, such as the empty promises of happiness from the people selling magical eating, the ignorant bidding of an un-woke medical establishment, and the belief that our bodies are not worthy of respect and love just as they are. Often we realize too late what we had. If you have ever looked back at old pictures of yourself and wondered why it was so difficult to see yourself as lovable and worthy, know that the body you have now is presenting you with a precious opportunity: to treat yourself with the love and care you wish you bestowed on your past self. The next time you have this experience, consider reading this contemplation by Traleg Kyabgon Rinpoche, author of *The Practice of Lojong: Cultivating Compassion through Training the Mind*: "If even mountains are subject to change and dissolution, how much more so is my own body, which is susceptible to disease, breakdown, the elements, accidents, and all kinds of harm? I must utilize my opportunities now, before that chance is lost forever."

How do you feel when you contemplate impermanence as it relates to your body?

The third preliminary—to recognize the cycle of karma: whatever you do has a result—relates to the cause-and-effect relationship between our states of mind, our actions, and our resulting experiences. This includes recognizing how thoughts give rise to emotions, which drive our actions, which affect our lives and the lives of those around us. This is how our thoughts create our world, for better and for worse. When we engage in actions that are good, the result is happiness. When we engage in actions that are damaging, the result is suffering. Whether an action is good or damaging is determined both by our intention and by how we affect ourselves and others. The ability to openly and honestly evaluate our intentions and the effects of our actions dictates the quality of our existence now and in the future.

Of course our very understanding of what is good and what is damaging has been deeply affected by magical eating, so getting to the bottom of how we perpetuate the cycle of karma through our thoughts and actions related to food and body is more complex. As a basic guide toward understanding what goodness means in terms of your thoughts or actions, and therefore your intentions, look to your own lived experience as the most valuable teacher. How has approaching food and your body according to the rules of magical eating affected the quality of your life? The quality of the lives of people around you?

There are two very different intentions behind anything we do for self-improvement: we are either problems that need to be fixed, or we accept ourselves as we are with compassion and the desire to be better. To the outside observer, these two intentions might look the same. Perhaps we attend our first yoga class or eat more fruits and vegetables. Only the individual herself knows the true intention motivating her changes in thoughts and behaviors. Viewing ourselves as problems to be fixed is a form of self-aggression (self-aggression that has become the cultural norm, but self-aggression nonetheless). Accepting ourselves with compassion and a desire to be better, on the other hand, is driven by belief in our basic goodness. Because the desire to be better comes from that place of basic okay-ness, it is much more sustainable.

It is this motivation that is perfectly captured by the Shunryu Suzuki Roshi quote, "Each of you is perfect the way you are... and you can use a little improvement." The story, as I recall, is that Suzuki Roshi was teaching some of his students at the San Francisco Zen Center in the 1970s and they were asking him questions about the path to enlightenment. How would they know if they were meditating correctly? How would they know how to interpret their insights? How would they be able to measure spiritual progress? Their questions were fueled by self-doubt and a clear desire to correct their inherent wrongness by doing things right. Their teacher saw through their lack of self-confidence and reassured them that they were indeed perfect, whole, and complete just as they were. At the same time, they could continue to become better. Though this seems a paradox, it is the most genuine way of relating to our complex and multifaceted selves. This ability to hold two seemingly conflicting points of view in the same heart is the basis of compassion.

Based on our sensory perceptions of sight, smell, taste, touch, and sound, our bodies are constantly communicating with us in the present moment. When we have thoughts and take actions aligned with this information, our intentions are good. Doing so also allows us to collect data that ultimately prove how our body's intelligence drives us toward actions that make us feel well, whole, and worthy. It is the collective effect of these experiences that prove our body's intrinsic wisdom. When we are not responding to our needs, on the other hand, our intentions aren't necessarily damaging or bad but likely confused. Because of the belief in basic goodness, the Buddhist tradition characterizes unsuccessful actions to be confused rather than bad. For example, if we eat past the point of satisfaction or comfortable fullness, it is not because our intentions are bad but because we are confused as to what our true needs are in the moment. Our confusion could be because we are resisting what our bodies are telling us or because we are ignorant to our body's communication. Confusion, if it is not recognized as such, always leads only to more confusion. But confusion that is acknowledged and worked with gently and compassionately may be transformed, and therefore our karma may be transformed.

The cycle of karma may also be considered in how our words and actions affect others. The ways in which we relate to our own bodies either perpetuate an unhealthy norm in our society or help disrupt it. By loudly voicing your criticisms of your body to be overheard by your children; bonding with others through diet talk, fat chat, or body bashing; or even commenting on others' bodies publicly or privately in a way that is not based on any true insight or understanding, we are only spreading the confusion of magical eating. Conversely, not fueling the fire of diet talk, changing the unending stream of media messages you consciously and unconsciously consume, and confidently inhabiting your body as you listen and respond to its needs will turn the tide of your personal body karma and model a different existence for those around you. Because magical eating is still considered so normal in our culture, disrupting it by intentionally defying its dysfunctional expectations, standards, and norms; nourishing yourself with kindness; and fully inhabiting the body you have may manifest as a radical form of activism. I will explain this further in chapter 6 on the paramita of exertion.

How do you feel when you contemplate the cycle of karma as it relates to your magical eating?

The fourth preliminary, to remember the unsatisfactory nature of suffering, defines suffering as an inevitable part of our lives. This runs counter to our culture's belief that suffering can be avoided if you just find the right *something*. But it is precisely the denial of this truth, the desire for suffering to be different than it is, that causes our suffering. This raises a concept in Buddhism called the first and second arrow. The first arrow is the inevitable suffering we all experience: impermanence and change, physical and emotional pain, illness, loss, and death. We have no control over the first arrow. The second arrow is how we respond to the first: with resistance, aggression, and gnashing of teeth, or with openness, warmth, and compassion. Unlike the first arrow, we do have some jurisdiction over the second. We either fight reality or accept it. When we fight it, we experience the suffering of suffering. When we accept it, we experience something else; it may not be pleasant, but it is genuine. By becoming aware of the first and second arrows in our lives and transforming how we respond, we become familiar with suffering as a natural part of life. This awareness may be used to cultivate compassion for ourselves and for others who suffer as well. When suffering is framed as workable, it becomes less scary. We are more apt to approach it with curiosity instead of fear.

Our suffering in terms of eating and our bodies is often due to a fundamental misunderstanding of our situation. We try to change who and how we are naturally in ways that only lead to more suffering. Much of our struggle stems from the belief that we should be able to sidestep pain, discomfort, and negative emotions by changing our bodies and controlling what we eat. But our bodies do not cause us to suffer; how we think about our bodies does. How we think about our bodies can also release us from suffering.

How do you feel when you contemplate the unsatisfactory nature of suffering?

By training in the preliminaries, we set the stage for a peaceful and sane relationship with food and our bodies. We are given one body with which to navigate our lives; how we relate to it affects everything and everyone we come into contact with. If we relate to our bodies with harsh restraint and fundamental unkindness, that is how we will be in the world. If we relate to our bodies with compassion and clear-seeing wisdom, that is what we will offer the world. Every moment presents us with the opportunity to go to sleep or to wake up, to harden or to soften, to live our lives in fear or in love.

3

THE PARAMITA

OF GENEROSITY

ENEROSITY IS A powerful place to begin because it comes from an internal desire to give and a willingness to let go. Generosity is often thought of as giving to others, but I would suggest true generosity begins with giving to ourselves. Chögyam Trungpa Rinpoche, the Tibetan meditation master who brought Shambhala Buddhism to the West, once said, "Generosity is a willingness to give, to open without philosophical or pious or religious motives, just simply doing what is required at any moment in any situation, not being afraid to receive anything." This suggests generosity is found in both giving and receiving.

When it is difficult for people to imagine being generous with others, one Buddhist practice involves passing an item from one hand to the other. I have always interpreted this as the need to give to oneself and to feel that one has enough before being generous with others. Enough may mean different things to different people and at different times, but essentially it is the confidence that our needs will be met. On the Eat to Love path, generosity begins with the willingness to recognize and meet our most basic needs of nourishment, water, rest, comfort, pleasure, and intimacy. Without judging or questioning, we are simply "doing what is required"; we sense what our basically good bodies need and do our best to give that to them. If we believe we are basically good and worthy of pleasure, satisfaction, and joy, we treat ourselves with the same generosity we extend to those we love.

There is much that remains unknown about how our bodies and our minds work. Even if science could prove that depriving our bodies of calories to lose weight was the key to unlocking better health (they haven't) or that eating clean was the route to a longer life (nope), very few people are able to do this in a sustainable way and instead wind up living with the harmful physical (weight cycling) and emotional (deprivation, feelings of failure) damage of diets. Rather than continuing the pursuit of elusive weight-loss methods, shouldn't we turn our search toward better ways to care for the bodies we have right now?

The industries selling magical eating got it backward. By teaching us that we are not inherently worthy of love and happiness and pleasure, they trained us to delay or deny ourselves the very things that could actually motivate us to take better care of ourselves. I can think of no better rationale for relying on the feedback from our own bodies and good judgment to care for ourselves as we are (rather than on all the constantly changing, or just plain wrong, information out there). A truly impressive body of scientific evidence has been accumulating to support this approach. Research continues to find that a non-diet or intuitive approach to eating and embodied movement, based on listening and responding to your unique body's wants, needs, and preferences, is the best approach to the care and feeding of yourself. In this chapter, you will learn how the senses guide us to connect with our innate intelligence and how shifting our allegiance to our internal sensations and away from the external cues that have distracted us from that intelligence is the very basis of generosity.

Becoming generous toward ourselves is disarming. When we feel vulnerable, we are taught to toughen our skin, but the world actually needs more willingness to experience that soft spot of vulnerability. In my experience, vulnerability begets vulnerability, and the heart-opening you feel elicits heart-opening in others, allowing us all to feel less alone. It is always important to recognize where you are in the process and what feels safe, to respect your personal edge. When you see where you are, you have choices you do not have when you don't see where you are. Once you recognize your limit, you might begin to experiment with opening up just a little more and to lean into that discomfort, knowing that there is much to be learned from it.

It is understandable if, after decades of magical eating and fighting with your body, it feels difficult or scary to maintain the open mind of generosity. Generosity toward ourselves may be thought of as selfish, gluttonous, or indulgent. Historically, depriving oneself of basic needs has even been associated with holiness. While thinness is not necessarily still conflated with holiness, there is some residual belief that eating and our bodies should be approached with restraint and that being generous toward ourselves is excessive and inappropriate. If you find treating yourself with generosity difficult at any point, simply notice it. Be gentle, and allow yourself to observe when doubts and fears arise. Try not to judge them as evidence that this path is not for you. See if you can practice generosity even toward your struggle to be generous.

Self-judgment is the greatest barrier to being generous with ourselves. We feel unworthy, whether inherently so or until we are able to change at some unknown future point. For this reason, it may be necessary to access a form of perception that exists before judgment in order to reconnect with our body's intelligence. With our senses of sight, hearing, smell, taste, and touch, our bodies experience the world outside and the world inside. Buddhists believe that enlightenment, the ability to see the true nature of reality, enters through the senses, which are always in the present moment, and that these are sharpened by a meditation practice. By connecting with the senses, we see things as they are, which is in and of itself a form of enlightenment. Our second lojong slogan (see page 61 for a reminder of what these are) emphasizes this point.

Examine the nature of unborn awareness

In this slogan, we transcend our judgments of good or bad and work with the purest nature of phenomena as they are. We examine unborn awareness primarily through the senses, what we feel, see, smell, hear, and taste, because these express reality unedited. In this space of raw perception, we are clear about what we feel without questioning ourselves. We are curious about our needs without judgment. And we respond to our body's requests without second-guessing. Acting on the unborn awareness of our senses also means giving ourselves absolute permission to eat what, when, and how much we want. (You will learn about this in greater detail later in the chapter.) This is not about swinging the pendulum from restraint to the other extreme. It is about continually removing barriers to discovering our true desires. Only without restriction may we begin to reveal our unique preferences.

Examining the nature of unborn awareness also means shifting our allegiance back from external things telling us what, when, and how much to eat to internal sensations of physical hunger and fullness, personal preference, and what we find satisfying. We nourish our bodies by valuing their intelligence, part of which is known as interoceptive awareness. Interoception includes feeling the sensations sent by our bodies and understanding them in real time: the awareness that we have to use the bathroom, that our heart is racing, that we are feeling hungry or becoming full. Meditation, with its emphasis on feeling, increases interoceptive awareness, including sensitivity to hunger and fullness sensations, and the ability to interpret them. This makes sense because meditation emphasizes being with our bodies as they are rather than trying to change anything. Our meditation practice is a direct and powerful support for our ability to examine the nature of unborn awareness. Feeling and understanding the information we receive from our bodies in real time allows us to respond in ways that are precise, balanced, and nourishing. Instead of overriding or changing our experience as we did with magical eating, we acknowledge what is actually happening more authentically, with honesty and curiosity, and respond to our true needs.

Before I go further into interoception and our internal sensations of physical hunger, fullness, preference, and satisfaction, let me first identify the many and varied external factors that tell us what, when, and how much to eat, if only so you can better recognize when you are *not* eating according to internal sensations.

External cues that tell us what to eat:

- "Eat this, not that" advice from doctors, dietitians, nutrition experts, and health coaches, or as read in traditional and social media
- Specific diet rules about what we should and should not eat (Paleo, vegan, raw, gluten-free, low-carb, low-fat, zero grams of sugar)

- Conscious or unconscious beliefs about foods being good or bad, healthy or unhealthy, virtuous or sinful
- Foods that seem appropriate in certain settings or situations (cereal for breakfast instead of salad, popcorn at a movie instead of shrimp cocktail)

External cues that tell us when to eat:

- Meal times (breakfast time, lunch time, snack time, dinner time, dessert time)
- Time of day (the moment we wake up, arriving at work, hitting the 3 p.m. slump, walking in the door after work, the moment we finish dinner, after the kids to go bed)
- The presence of food even if we're not hungry (food leftover from a meeting in the conference room, the dessert tray appearing after an already satisfying meal, the availability of novel foods while staying at a friend's house)
- Other people encouraging us to eat ("You're going to make me eat alone?" or "You have to try this!")
- Situations in which eating feels obligatory (work functions, family meals, bagel Fridays, pizza Mondays, birthday cake celebrations, free food offered as a pseudo-perk)
- Situational triggers (sitting in front of the TV, watching a movie, attending a sporting event, or being on a long drive)
- Emotional triggers (anger, sadness, loneliness, stress, happiness, or boredom)

External cues that tell us how much to eat:

- Package sizes
- Serving sizes as listed on nutrition labels
- Round numbers (10 chips, 20 almonds, etc.)
- How much we are served, and whether we are served by ourselves or by someone else
- Number of calories, points, exchanges, or grams of sugar, carbohydrates, protein, fat, or fiber in a particular food
- The amount eaten by other people
- The amount of food left in a package, carton, bag, or on a plate

- Certain situational triggers (sitting in front of the TV, getting too hungry, drinking alcohol, smoking marijuana)

It is completely normal for our eating to sometimes be influenced by external cues. Part of shifting our allegiance to our own intelligence means understanding and respecting our personal preferences, which may be influenced by situations and circumstances like those I just listed. That said, with the Eat to Love approach, the primary driver for your eating is what you feel, otherwise described as your internal experience of hunger, fullness, preference, and satisfaction. Your internal cues are the physical sensations you experience by being fully in your body.

Let's examine the feelings associated with hunger and fullness. How hunger and fullness feel in our bodies is as unique as we are. The sample hunger and fullness scales below, in which I use the numbers one through ten, descriptive words, and sensory and experiential explanations, express what hunger and fullness feel like for *me* specifically.

Personalized Hunger Scale

Hunger level	Number	Sensory/experiential descriptors
Not Hungry	1	Absence of hunger sensations, mouth feels neutral
Gently hungry	2–3	Feeling of emptiness in the stomach, slight rumbling in stomach, early hunger pangs
Hungry	4–5	Stomach churning, stronger hunger pangs, slight discomfort in stomach, thinking about food
Very hungry	6–7	Uncomfortable churning in the stomach, slight pain in upper abdomen, preoccupation with my mouth, unable to concentrate
Ravenous	8–9	Irritable, headache, jaw clenched, stomach sensations might temporarily abate
Painfully hungry	10	"Hangry," painful sensation in the upper stomach behind my ribcage

Personalized Fullness Scale

Fullness level	Number	Sensory/experiential descriptors
Not full at all	1	Absence of fullness sensations, stomach feels neutral
No longer hungry	2–3	Sense that hunger has decreased or is absent but not yet feeling distention in stomach, stomach might feel a pleasant weight, could still comfortably eat
Slightly full	4	Slight distention in the stomach, food starts to taste less delicious, nearing satisfaction
Comfortably full	5–6	Greater distention in the stomach but not uncomfortable, feels like *enough* in the body, less drive to put food in my mouth
Very full	7–8	Stomach distention begins to feel uncomfortable, clothing begins to pull and feel tight against my stomach and skin, food in my mouth actually feels unpleasant
Stuffed	9	Very uncomfortable, slight sense of reflux, sluggish
Sick	10	Extremely uncomfortable, nauseated, need to lie down

By familiarizing ourselves with our unique experience of hunger and fullness, we are able to identify how hungry we prefer to be when we begin eating and how full we prefer to be when we stop. I think of hunger and fullness as an ongoing conversation we have with our bodies. When the body first starts to get hungry, it lets you know with a whisper. A feeling of emptiness in your stomach is like your body softly saying, *We should probably start thinking about what we're going to have for lunch.* After a little time has passed, the sensation gets stronger; perhaps there's audible grumbling, and the conversation gets a little louder. *It's that time. You're listening, right? I need some energy!* And if we do not respond, it is not long before the sensation ventures into the really uncomfortable, and the conversation escalates to a much higher volume. *HELLO???* *STOP WHAT YOU'RE DOING. NOW.*

The type of eating experience we have depends a lot on when in the course of this conversation we respond to our body's needs. For example, if we were to start eating somewhere between the first and second signals above, which might be described as gently hungry or hungry, we are more likely to sense what we are hungry for in that particular moment, to eat at a pace that is compatible with enjoyment, and to notice as the physical sensations of fullness emerge. On the other hand, if we wait until the third, ALL CAPS portion of the conversation, we are less likely to know what we are hungry for and might desire different foods than if we responded earlier, for example, high-carbohydrate snacks to quickly regulate tanking blood sugar levels. We are also more likely to eat faster, potentially decreasing our enjoyment of the meal and our awareness of emerging fullness, and to eat past the point of comfortable fullness.

Many of us have had the experience where we get super hungry, but for one reason or another we do not pause to eat, only to find that the physical sensations seem to disappear. Whether we intentionally skipped a meal or could not tear ourselves away from working on a looming deadline, we might mistake this for the disappearance of our hunger. Let me assure you, this does not mean that your body is no longer hungry. I lack the typographical power to one-up ALL CAPS so instead think of this as being similar to what happens when someone is vehemently demanding your attention and you fail to give it; perhaps they quiet down for a moment, walk into the kitchen, and search for some pots and pans to bang together. When they return, They. Mean. Business. And it is the same with our hunger; when we ignore it, it comes back with a vengeance. As it should! When we get this hungry, we are more likely to overeat at our next meal, as well as at subsequent meals. Eating in this way may feel frenetic, out of control, and very much like emotional overeating. I will discuss emotional overeating in the next chapter on the paramita of discipline, but when working toward ending emotional overeating, it is extremely important to differentiate it from getting too hungry, to recognize and respond to the body's physical hunger sensations appropriately so that we are eating satisfyingly and consistently throughout the day instead of in this chaotic way.

Continuing with the conversation analogy, the sensations associated with various degrees of fullness begin with a whisper and culminate in a howl. The continuum of fullness goes from the point at which we no longer feel hungry—that is, the sensation is the absence of hunger—through the shades of gray often communicated by a growing sensation of physical distention or stretch in the stomach, all the way up to the point at which we are really uncomfortable or even experience reflux-like symptoms, nausea, or pain.

One of the earliest physical sensations of emerging fullness is that the food we are eating starts to taste a little less spectacular. This connection between how good food tastes and how hungry we are is an evolutionary feature that drives us to eat when we need food and to stop when we have had enough. If we pay attention to how a food tastes as we eat it, we might notice there is a marked difference between bite one and bite twenty. But sometimes we just want to keep on eating. Perhaps you have observed this when dining with a group of people; after a few minutes of eating the body begins to become satisfied and to decrease the taste rewards it sends to the brain. But if the food is delicious and the general atmosphere is enjoyable, people might want to continue eating despite this diminishing return. Desiring to experience the same high taste reward they had at the beginning of the meal, many people reach for the salt shaker, to boost the brain's perception of the food's flavor.

When we first consider physical hunger and fullness, we might think we have only two extreme settings, starving and stuffed, with brief moments of not hungry/not full somewhere in the middle. However, just as a gas tank is rarely squarely on Empty or Full, our bodies register many gradients of hunger and fullness between the extremes of starving and stuffed. In addition, hunger and fullness do not necessarily exist on one continuum. It is possible to feel somewhat full and to still feel hungry. This is why the two scales are separated and should be considered at the same time, but not as one. As we begin to place our awareness on the physical sensations of hunger and fullness, we notice what those shades of gray feel like in our unique bodies.

Begin to identify the levels of hunger and fullness associated with your most enjoyable eating experience using the following hunger and fullness scales to define what the various points in the scales feel like in your body. On the hunger scale, the number 1 signifies the absence of hunger while 10 signifies the hungriest your body has ever felt. Similarly, on the fullness scale, 1 signifies the absence of fullness while 10 signifies the fullest you have ever felt.

Your Hunger Scale

Hunger level	Number	Sensory/experiential descriptors
Not hungry	1	
Gently hungry	2–3	
Hungry	4–5	
Very hungry	6–7	
Ravenous	8–9	
Painfully hungry	10	

Your Fullness Scale

Fullness level	Number	Sensory/experiential descriptors
Not full at all	1	
No longer hungry	2–3	
Slightly full	4	
Comfortably full	5–6	
Very full	7–8	
Stuffed	9	
Sick	10	

By becoming more familiar with the physical sensations of hunger and fullness, we avoid the extremes. By feeding ourselves consistently and satisfyingly, we are relieved of the physical discomfort of extreme hunger and fullness. Such extremes act as a stress on the body, yet many of us with a history of magical eating do not feel we deserve to eat until our hunger is very intense. By examining the nature of unborn awareness, we respond to our bodies earlier in the "conversation," when they ask to be fed; we eat regularly throughout the day and generally do not go longer than about four hours without eating something.

Becoming familiar with the full spectrum of your physical hunger allows you to eventually identify the level of hunger that is most compatible with an enjoyable eating experience. For most people, this means feeling enough hunger that food tastes good but not such a high level of hunger that you feel out of control when you finally begin to eat. This is your *middle way* of hunger, not too little and not too much. Similarly, you will be able to identify the degree of fullness most comfortable for you. You might eat smaller meals more frequently throughout the day and therefore eat to a lesser degree of fullness, no longer hungry or slightly full. By eating to a lesser degree of fullness, you are likely to become hungry again sooner. Or you might prefer to eat three meals a day and not to snack, eating to a greater degree of fullness on most occasions, such as to the point of comfortably full or even very full. By eating to this greater degree of fullness, you are more likely to go a longer period of time before feeling hungry again.

Different situations might also prompt adjustments to how you eat. If you notice you are hungry an hour before a special dinner at a restaurant, you could choose to eat something on the lighter side, to the point of feeling no longer hungry, so that you are your desired level of hungry when you arrive at the restaurant. Or, if you have an afternoon packed with meetings and do not anticipate the opportunity to eat again, you could choose to eat lunch to a greater degree of fullness to sustain yourself for the hours ahead. Though many of us have typical patterns in terms of how we eat—smaller, more frequent meals or fewer, larger meals—the Eat to Love approach involves being receptive to your body's changing needs so that what, when, how much, and generally how you eat varies based on your specific needs at the time. Flexibility is key.

When we eat according to internal sensations, consistently and over time, our body weight normalizes. It naturally finds the range at which it is most comfortable, without our needing to exert extreme control over it. Whether that range is higher or lower than your current one is determined by your body's unique characteristics and experiences. As we touched on before, bodies come in all different shapes and sizes. Your natural weight is the one you can sustain without struggle, chaos, or deprivation.

When you eat regularly throughout the day and discover your middle way of hunger and fullness, you might also notice some change in your overall approach to eating. Many of my clients who began by eating in a very restrained way throughout the day and then overate at night have found that eating regularly throughout the day decreases the physical and emotional experiences that used to trigger nighttime overeating. Some have experienced a decreased need for stimulants like coffee, tea, or soda and a lesser preference for high-sugar foods between meals because their bodies are able to maintain balanced blood sugar levels throughout the day. If you have had a history of deprivation, beginning to eat regularly may at first feel like you are always eating, but please know that with time this will normalize. Trust your body to guide you toward what you need.

As you examine your feelings and experiences, here are some questions that can help you begin to connect the dots between the hunger level at which you eat and the resulting eating event.

Contemplate what your eating experience is like when you begin eating at a hunger level between 1 and 3, between 4 and 7, or between 8 and 10. How well do you know what you are hungry for when you begin eating at these different hunger levels? How fast do you eat? How good does the food taste and how enjoyable is the overall eating experience? What level of fullness do you tend to eat to?

What do you think your middle way of hunger and fullness is? Why is it generous to respect your own middle way?

In examining the nature of unborn awareness through familiarization with the physical sensations of hunger and fullness, we notice how concepts, beliefs, and judgments interfere with responding genuinely. As we pay more attention to the internal environment, we start to notice how they contradict deeply held concepts in our minds (usually externally driven concepts). How many times have you had the following thoughts?

- I shouldn't be hungry, I ate an hour ago.
- It's lunchtime, I should eat something.
- I'm hungry for carbs / chocolate / something salty, but I shouldn't eat it.
- I'm still hungry but I've already eaten a serving; I shouldn't eat any more.
- I'm full but there's food left on my plate; I might as well finish it.

While the sensations of hunger and fullness are internal physical experiences unique to your body, which suggests you are in fact the best judge of what, when, and how much to eat, at times you might have a greater allegiance to some external determinant. This is not a problem. Noticing the dissonance is a normal part of shifting your allegiance. Noticing when you feel pulled to behave in specific ways by external factors is an essential part of this process. It is also important to notice how a greater allegiance to external cues causes us to eat when we are not hungry, such as in the case of a mealtime arriving even though we are not experiencing hunger yet, or not to eat when we are hungry, as when we get hungry at 11 a.m. but it is not lunchtime yet.

What are the external cues that most frequently get in the way of listening to your internal hunger and fullness sensations? How can you consciously shift your allegiance back to internal sensations in these moments?

Not only does examining the nature of unborn awareness help us have the most comfortable eating experience, it also guides us to eat for the greatest nourishment and enjoyment. Though there is very little scientific evidence supporting the importance of pleasure from a nutrition standpoint, one study that emerged in the late 1970s showed that how much a meal was enjoyed could affect how nutrients were absorbed. Researchers from Thailand and Sweden collaborated to examine whether cultural food preferences affected how iron was absorbed. In the first phase of the study, Thai and Swedish women were served a typical Thai dish of rice, vegetables, coconut, and hot chili paste. The dish was generally more enjoyed by the Thai women, who also absorbed twice as much iron as the Swedish women (who enjoyed the meal less). When served a traditional Swedish dish of hamburger, mashed potatoes, and string beans, the Swedish women absorbed more iron than the Thai women. In the second phase of the study, participants were placed in subgroups; half the women were given traditional Thai or Swedish meals while the other half were served the same meals that had been puréed into a mush so that it was less enjoyable. Women served the less enjoyable version of the meal, though it contained the exact same amounts of nutrients, absorbed significantly lower amounts of iron. Not that we need an argument against the pillification of eating, but this suggests "you are *how* you eat." Enjoyment of what we eat matters whether or not it affects how much of the nutrients we absorb. The joy of eating is one of the simplest pleasures in life, connecting us to our own basic goodness and the goodness of others.

A simple means of connecting with the joy of eating is a mindful eating practice. Mindful eating has roots in a Zen Buddhist tradition called oryoki, translated as *just enough*. Oryoki is still practiced as a group in meditation retreats and consists of efficient and choreographed steps in which participants serve themselves, eat silently, and clean up, all while placing their full attention on the task at hand. Oryoki emphasizes focusing on a single activity, taking our time, and appreciating the full depth and breadth of eating with our bodies. Though oryoki practice is a personal one that each individual does alone (even when practiced in a room with many other people), it has broader implications. Such a simple practice involves narrowing our focus to do one thing at a time. Slowing down and connecting with the raw perception of sight, sound, smell, taste, and texture facilitates shifting our allegiance from the torrent of external things telling us how to eat and care for ourselves to an inner wisdom. Beyond that, a mindful eating or oryoki-like practice allows us to sit in silence (with or without others) and appreciate our connection with others, whether with those sitting beside us or those who grew the food, transported it, and prepared it.

A classic mindful eating exercise involves eating a single raisin: examining it with your eyes, fingers, and nose before placing it in your mouth, and savoring it in slow motion before chewing and then swallowing it. But most of us are moving at such a fast pace that we race through our meals and find it difficult to imagine taking pleasure in a single raisin. A mindful eating practice need not be painstaking. As with all aspects of this path, choose what feels most meaningful to you.

ONE OF MY first clients, Pina, came to me because she couldn't stop eating handfuls of peanut M&Ms from the bowl on her secretary's desk when the clock hit 3 p.m. We decided to do a mindful eating exercise with peanut M&Ms in which we slowed things down and ate them one at a time. As she raised the first peanut M&M to her eyes, Pina remarked that it was the first time she'd ever really looked at one. She noticed tiny cracks in the candy shell, how each was differently shaped, and how her mouth watered with the anticipation of eating. But as she slowly ate one of them she realized, to her initial dismay, that she didn't really enjoy it. When she ate them by the handful, she had been driven by extreme hunger and an emotional need for a break. The impact of a handful of peanut M&Ms had been so overwhelming to her senses of taste and touch (texture) that it obscured the fact that, taken one at a time, they weren't even pleasing to her palate. As a result of that experiment, Pina decided to eat a more satisfying lunch, to have substantial snacks on hand when hunger naturally hit mid-afternoon, to have alternative ways of taking a break if she wasn't hungry, and to stock high-quality chocolate-covered nuts and fruit in her own desk for when that specific craving arose.

Eating with the senses begins by choosing foods that please the eye, the nose, the palate (in terms of taste and texture), and even the ear. Emphasizing the sensual aspects of appearance, aroma, taste, and texture and truly savoring what you are eating synchronizes your mind with your body. Doing so allows you to notice what your actual experience is and how it changes from one moment to the next. You might observe, for example, that you have fairly specific preferences in terms of the temperature at which food is served, the exact balance of spices, particular tastes at distinct times of the day or year, favorite textures, filling capacities, and quality of ingredients. You might even detect that those foods you thought were favorites are not what you imagined, while others emerge as particularly satisfying and enjoyable.

Chefs are fond of saying we eat with our eyes first. This is because we usually look at food before we taste it. Choosing foods that please the eye enhances our satisfaction by connecting us with the food's inherent beauty. By extension, consuming beautiful, high-quality foods (which need not be expensive) makes us feel we are caring for ourselves. This is inherently generous. Eventually we discern the difference between feeding physical hunger in ways that please the eye and eating when we are not hungry because we are triggered by the sight of something enticing. With continued attention and practice, you might reach a point at which you appreciate and feel satisfied by the simple sight of beautiful foods, even if you do not happen to be hungry at the moment you see them. It may be difficult to imagine enjoying beautiful pastries in a shop window without eating them, but once you have felt the connection that foods taste best when you are both physically hungry and when you have a specific craving for them, you might admire a food's beauty even if you are not going to eat it right then. Not that you cannot eat when you are not hungry. With absolute permission, eating is always an option. This is a subtle but important point. There is no right or wrong choice in this situation; there is only *your* choice and the resulting experience to learn from. Being on your own Eat to Love path means choosing what feels good to you, based on your own set of criteria. When you are used to eating on autopilot, the freedom of choice makes all the difference.

Just as we choose foods that are beautiful to look at, the aromas, tastes, and textures of our food contribute to a unique sensory eating experience and level of enjoyment. Again there is a difference between appreciating the smells, tastes, and textures of foods when we are feeding our physical hunger and being triggered by a certain smell or the desire for a specific taste or texture in our mouths when we are not physically hungry. By practicing with noticing our desires, whims, cravings, and tastes, and reinforcing the idea that we have absolute permission to eat what, when, and how much we truly desire, we become more and more able to respond to our actual needs skillfully and precisely (rather than reacting automatically). Sometimes we just want something crunchy, salty, creamy, or fatty in our mouths regardless of physical hunger. Other times we find that no amount of the food we momentarily crave will satisfy our true desires. I will go into the emotional side of eating in greater detail in the next chapter on the paramita of discipline.

As I touched on above, a food's taste changes as we eat and as our bodies become satisfied because our brains perceive the taste of the food as less and less delicious.

ANDREA NOTICED A change in her perception of a favorite food one night as she was eating a bowl of hazelnut gelato after dinner. We had been working together for several months and had discussed this concept but also talked about how she shouldn't rush it. She would get there when she got there. When Andrea came in for a session one day, she shared that the night before, while enjoying her gelato with all of her senses, she discovered a clear difference between bite nine and bite ten and decided to stop there. She recognized she had reached the mysterious point of enough. When she began, Andrea decided that the most generous thing was to eat the gelato she craved, while at the point she realized she'd had enough, she knew that true generosity for her meant stopping precisely when she did.

As much as our sense of touch in terms of texture deepens our connection with food, engaging with food chosen by our own hands has much the same effect. Many clients describe a greater sense of satisfaction when they pick their own ingredients, prepare some of their own meals and snacks, and cook, even if it is not something out of *Gourmet* magazine. Just like choosing ingredients and foods of the highest quality you can afford, engaging with food through preparation and cooking feels like a form of self-care, which makes the process more satisfying and enjoyable. Compared with beginning to engage with food when we open the door to the pizza delivery guy, taking the time to make the dough and prepare the ingredients makes a homemade pizza more satisfying. That said, please order take-out whenever you wish. The point is to experiment with various choices and begin to gain an understanding of what would give you the most pleasure. With time and practice, this form of paying attention translates into the ability to decipher what would be most enjoyable from one situation to the next.

Perhaps one of the best-known aspects of eating with the senses relates to slowing down the pace of eating. This may mean different things to different people at different times. For you, slowing down might mean making time for meals rather than skipping them, sitting down rather than eating on the run or standing over the sink, or removing distractions such as the television and other electronic devices. Or it may mean eating the first five or ten minutes of a meal in silence in order to focus your attention primarily on the sensuality of the food. Taking just one bite with attention and intention brings you into the present moment and connects you with food and your body in a meaningful way. It is the connection with the sense perceptions, and therefore our bodies, that allows us to feel what is actually happening with precision, openness, and curiosity. An added benefit: being in the moment enhances our enjoyment!

By bringing generosity into our relationship with food and our bodies by connecting with the pre-conceptual, pre-judgment perception of our senses, we begin to amass evidence that our bodies can be trusted. With each experience in which the intelligence of our bodies leads us to eat in a way that is pleasurable, satisfying, and aligned with our appetites, we gain confidence and connection with our unique Eat to Love path. As we gain this confidence and trust in our bodies and our judgment, we are free to practice generosity more fully.

In Buddhist thought, there are three types of generosity: ordinary, fearlessness, and the gift of dharma. Ordinary generosity consists of taking care of ourselves and others, providing comfort in the form of goods and acts of service, and treating ourselves and others with gentleness. Fearlessness, the second form of generosity, involves leaping onto this path even if you don't feel 100 percent sure or ready and tolerating a degree of uncertainty while trusting in the process. With fearlessness, you begin to turn your generosity practice outward, in how your present yourself to the world, how you speak about your body and all bodies, and the ways in which you shift the language and conversations of magical eating toward something more beneficial. The third form of generosity is sharing the dharma, or the truth about the tolls of magical eating and self-aggression, with others. This opens their eyes to a new way of supporting you on your path and may help them to relate differently to their own bodies.

Our meditation practice could be thought of as all three forms of generosity. It is a form of ordinary generosity and caregiving in that we allow ourselves to be as we are, without aggression and without agenda. It is fearless to pause in the midst of our crazed world of endless doing to feel what is arising in the moment. And it is sharing the dharma even if you never utter a word about your practice, because the ways in which you extend into the world around you are influenced by the stability and openness gained from meditating.

1. Ordinary Generosity

Satisfaction

Practicing ordinary generosity toward ourselves includes making satisfaction a priority. Satisfaction exists on two levels: physical and psychological. Physical satisfaction is what happens when you eat enough energy for your body; it is meeting a need in a very functional way by eating the three macronutrients: carbohydrates, protein, and fat. The three macronutrients are satisfying to the body in different ways (something I will go into in more depth in the chapter on the paramita of wisdom). However, the satisfaction you get from eating the amount of carbohydrates, protein, and fat your body needs is different from the satisfaction you get from eating the food your body (and mind and heart) craves. Have you ever had the experience of eating something that satisfied you physically but not psychologically, so that even though you were comfortably full, you found yourself longing for something more? Perhaps you found yourself unsatisfied after eating "heavy pupu" at a cocktail party because you were hungry for a full sit-down meal or after a meal of broiled salmon and steamed broccoli when you really wanted the pasta. The additional layer of psychological (or emotional) satisfaction comes from eating what and how you want to eat, whether because of sensory characteristics such as appearance, aroma, taste, texture, temperature, and filling capacity; pleasant associations from your past experiences; or simply being in the moment and connecting with the senses.

Intuitive Eating, a scientifically validated model created by registered dietitians Evelyn Tribole and Elyse Resch, first positioned satisfaction as the "driving force" of eating according to internal sensations. As a result of their decades of work in healing unpeaceful eating, Tribole and Resch place satisfaction at the center of the other Intuitive Eating principles. This is because a true sense of satisfaction, based on eating exactly what you want, when you want it, and in the exact amount that feels like enough, is essential to a peaceful and sustainable relationship with food. The key to understanding what satisfies you psychologically is giving yourself absolute permission to eat and viewing all foods on an equal moral plane. This means the carrot and the carrot cake are both just foods with different amounts of carbohydrates, protein, and fat. One is not inherently better or worse, more or less healthful, than the other. Only with absolute permission to eat do you really start to understand what you're hungry for, why, and how much you need to feel like you've eaten enough. Or, as my client Patricia put it, "Only after I stopped trying to control everything I ate did I finally feel in control."

I often ask my clients how they would eat if satisfaction were the ultimate goal. At first, they respond that eating the foods they have always forbidden themselves would contribute to the greatest satisfaction. Cakes, cookies, ice cream, candy, chocolate, pastries, pizza, take-out, and fast food rank high on the list. The desire for the things we aren't supposed to want cannot be underestimated. I experienced this firsthand while pregnant when I was advised not to eat ripened cheeses and deli meats due to the risk of foodborne illness. Normally I couldn't care less about these foods, but what do you think I craved during my pregnancy? Blue cheese and sliced turkey, simply because I wasn't supposed to have them.

What happens when we don't give ourselves absolute permission to eat is that we start to compensate for it in different ways. When you don't want to give in to a food craving and instead substitute a "safer" option, you are likely to eat more of that food than you actually need to physically satisfy you. (Beware of anyone peddling "mindful substitutions" for this reason.) This tendency to make up for the lack of quality in eating with greater quantity of a less satisfying food is chasing the satisfaction you would have gotten from just eating what you originally desired. Even after eating too much of an unsatisfying substitute, many clients (and I too in the past) go on to eat what they initially craved to finally hit that sweet spot of satisfaction. But they end up missing the mark; no longer being hungry and having eaten too much overall dampens the reward of eventually eating what you first craved. In this situation, the wise and generous decision would have been to eat what you really wanted, to be present with and undistracted from the eating, and to give yourself permission to fully enjoy it.

During our work together, my clients begin to give themselves absolute permission to eat what they want, especially those things they formerly restricted. They also continue to eat the foods they previously considered safe but with a different kind of attention. The result is that they start to learn what they actually like. In many cases, this includes realizing that those forbidden foods they thought they always craved really weren't all that and a bag of chips. Or they discover that they do like those foods but only in certain circumstances, quantities, or from specific, high-quality brands. Alternatively many people realize that the foods they ate out of a sense of duty because they were supposedly safe or healthy were not their favorites, and they give themselves permission not to eat them. Or they realize they really do like them and therefore continue to eat them, but with enjoyment rather than obligation.

WHEN WE STARTED working together, Melissa was convinced her body was different from the bodies of other people I had worked with. She believed that hers simply could not be trusted to guide her toward a varied diet and that, if left to her own devices, she would eat cheeseburgers, fries, and chocolate milkshakes from morning till night. "Try it," I advised her. We worked to give her absolute permission to eat what she really wanted. When she finally agreed, the craving for cheeseburgers lasted half a day. On her way home from work, Melissa spied some fresh summer peaches for sale at a fruit stand and realized they were what she was really hungry for in the moment. The idea that her body could tell her what to eat and that it would drive her toward a varied and balanced diet seemed too good to be true. Melissa had to prove it to herself.

Restriction, whether real or imagined, self-imposed or otherwise, provokes rebellion. Removing the restriction removes the need to rebel. This is an act of true generosity; it is when the process of understanding what you truly like begins. In addition to affecting what you choose to eat, giving yourself absolute permission affects how much you need to eat to feel you have reached the point of enough. Again, at the beginning of working together, clients often assume that eating more will contribute to a greater sense of satisfaction. Once they have given themselves permission to have as much as they truly want in any given situation, the allure of more starts to fade and they find that how much they need to feel satisfied is nuanced. Sometimes more is just more and doesn't equate with greater satisfaction. Other times more is actually what they need because their bodies are hungrier.

Other contributors to satisfaction include food values. Food values are principles that guide your eating because of their impact on other beings. These are important considerations and represent some of the ways in which our relationship with food and eating is inherently emotional (and that is a good thing!). Occasionally, however, our food values conflict with our internal physical sensations of hunger and fullness. When this is the case, you must choose what to prioritize, knowing that there is no right or wrong answer, just choices to reflect upon and potentially make differently in the future. On occasion, magical eating could be masquerading as a food value. Only you will truly know what is what in these situations, so it is important to be honest with yourself about your real intentions.

One common food value many people grew up with was not wasting food out of respect for the food itself, the money spent on it, and those who live with food insecurity. If not wasting food is a food value for you (including taking advantage of free food), you might consider how to work with it and still respect your internal sensations of hunger and fullness. Eating more than you need to feel satisfied may not be your only option. Freezing food, donating it, or composting may all allow you to respect your body's internal signals as well as your food values.

Similarly, some people value eating local or organic meat and produce, or prioritizing seasonal eating. If these are food values for you, pay attention to whether eating according to this standard ever contributes to feelings of deprivation (from not being allowed to eat the things that don't meet these standards) or guilt or remorse (for having allowed yourself to eat such foods). A fixation on "eating healthy" is a form of disordered eating unto its own, known as orthorexia, and should be acknowledged if obsession with health actually begins to detract from it. Supporting organic, local, and seasonal growers and purveyors is one way of eating according to your values, and it may also be done in a good enough way so that it doesn't have to be black and white.

The same could be said for the food value of eating vegan or vegetarian. Choosing to eat in these ways, for ethical reasons, is an important expression of your values, but if you are not able to meet your nutritional needs or experience deprivation, consider a middle way. I do believe it is possible to decrease the overall suffering of beings by choosing carefully who we purchase eggs, dairy, and meats from based on how the animals are treated, the conditions in which they live, and the ways in which the products we ultimately consume are obtained. Each of our bodies is unique; recognizing whether a vegan or vegetarian diet truly works for you is a form of honesty and generosity.

Another food value is eating more frequently solely as a form of entertainment and pleasure. If you value eating more frequently for pleasure, meaning eating often in the absence of physical hunger, you could find that this leads to a higher natural weight range. You may also choose whether to eat to fuel your athletic performance or to place more or less value on the wellness potentially gained through eating and activity behaviors. Basically, any choice you make that may seem to agree or conflict with our cultural norms, standards, and expectations around health, eating, weight, and body image may be your personal food value.

Taking the leap of listening to and trusting our bodies to tell us what, when, and how much to eat leads us to discover that what is truly satisfying includes a variety of foods in different amounts, and that this changes from day to day, month to month, and year to year.

What, when, how much, and generally how would you eat if satisfaction were your highest priority? What are your food values? Do they ever conflict with respecting your internal sensations of hunger and fullness? How can you reconcile this disconnect most generously?

Comfort and Pleasure

The austerity of the diet culture suggests we do not deserve comfort and physical pleasure until our bodies comply with the narrow standards it created. In the Eat to Love approach, you deserve comfort and physical pleasure simply because you exist and are basically good. By now we understand that self-aggression and restraint are not motivating. Delaying treating ourselves with kindness will always be a carrot-and-stick situation. Treating ourselves and our bodies with generosity is inherently more motivating. We take better care of what we love. And we love what we take good care of. It is possible to show ourselves this love by respecting our basic needs for comfort, touch, sensuality, and pleasure. Denying ourselves this or constantly delaying our gratification is denying our basic humanity.

As I explained above, avoiding the discomfort of extreme hunger and fullness is a good start toward giving yourself more comfort. Another way is to drink enough water by giving yourself permission to not experience the discomfort of being chronically dehydrated. If you are someone who struggles to drink enough water, try experimenting with your water preferences and what encourages you to drink according to your true needs. Do you like it cold or room temperature? Fizzy or flat? Full glasses at a time, or small sips throughout the day? What type of glass do you most enjoy drinking from? Do you prefer to drink from a personal water bottle? If you prefer a water bottle, what type of spout? A straw you suck through, the type of straw you have to bite and suck, a drinking spout, or from the edge, like drinking from a cup? Notice any associations you have with drinking water, which may include magical eating thoughts that drinking water curbs hunger and tricks your body into eating less. Yet we all need to drink water, so why not do it in a way that is pleasurable?

Other ways to increase comfort include giving yourself permission to opt out of the discomfort of many overlooked basic items, such as underwear, bras, pantyhose, and camisoles. You deserve to wear underwear that is not frayed, holey, or threadbare; that does not bunch up or roll down. You deserve bras that do not dig into your shoulders or under your arms, that support your breasts comfortably without pain. You deserve pantyhose and tights that don't roll down, cut off your circulation, or squeeze your belly or thighs, and camisoles that don't roll up or constrict your torso. Despite the vigor with which shapewear is sold to women, you have a choice of comfort over camouflage.

Giving yourself greater comfort might also mean letting go of "aspirational" clothes, those that no longer fit but that you hang on to just in case, and replacing them with shirts that button comfortably, sweaters that fit as you like, pants that move with you, and skirts and dresses that feel comfortable on your body no matter what the arbitrarily determined size on the little tag says. When choosing these clothes, select fabrics that feel good against your skin, that allow your body to be at its ideal temperature, and that let your body walk, sit, and eat comfortably. You could also give yourself permission to have furniture that fits and supports your body, that allows you to feel comfortable and welcomed. The spaces in which you live, work, and rest could similarly be made more comfortable and welcoming. When you begin to consider ways in which to give yourself physical comfort, it may be surprising how much discomfort you have been tolerating.

Putting my son to bed one night when he had a bad cold, I was struck by how intuitive our sensuality is. As I was rubbing his head (and every time I stopped, he dragged my hand back to it), he simultaneously sucked on his pacifier, cuddled his oh-so-soft woo-woo, and rubbed his palm back and forth across the sheet. Our need for touch and care is inherent in having senses. We crave this sort of physical stimulation and pleasure. Maybe we could survive without it, but why?

Increasing physical pleasure could be as simple as taking a shower or bath at the exact temperature you love, using bath products that smell gorgeous and that soothe your hair and skin, wrapping yourself in the softest towel, and putting lotion or scented oils on your hands and body. Lying down in the most luxurious sheets, or cuddling in the coziest blankets. Getting your hair done; getting a massage, foot rub, or head rub; getting or giving yourself a manicure and pedicure; getting or giving yourself a facial or body scrub. Though many are limited by financial resources and access, some of the simplest things can provide pleasure, such as watching a favorite movie or TV show. Listening to music that fills your heart with joy (or sadness, or longing, if that's your thing). Viewing art that gets your heart beating faster or sets your imagination in motion. Attending a theater production, musical, ballet, or opera that transports you emotionally. Spending time with people who uplift you and allowing yourself to be in environments that feel welcoming, joyous, or fulfilling, such as in nature, at a museum, at a concert, or curling up on the couch with a book.

JILL GREW UP in a strict religious community that was controlling of women's bodies and judgmental about how they should be dressed. Physical pleasure from sensuality, sexuality, and even socializing with men was associated with wrongdoing. At the same time, her community confusingly emphasized the physical beauty of women and an abundance and variety of foods, particularly during the holidays, which seemed to happen every other weekend. Jill grew up fairly comfortable with her non-skinny body until she reached puberty, at which time the scrutiny of her community felt oppressive. From her sisters, cousins, and aunts, she learned which foods were good and which were bad for weight control. Jill came to see me years after leaving the community from which she learned to fear pleasure. At that time, she had gained weight and often found herself eating very quickly. "Bad" foods were eaten with a sense of "getting it over with"; "good" foods were eaten quickly because they were not meant to be enjoyed. She also continued to struggle with whether she deserved to eat, to be in her body, and to enjoy sensual pleasures. After several sessions discussing the basic human need for pleasure and sensuality, not only was Jill able to derive enjoyment from the foods she chose to eat and to slow down the pace of her eating, she gave herself permission to experience physical pleasure from massage, from taking leisurely walks in the city with no destination in mind, and in meeting up regularly with friends who filled her heart with joy (even after overeating, which, in the past, would have caused her to cancel plans and cocoon at home).

Bringing embodied movement back into your life is another form of comfort and pleasure. Your relationship with physical activity might have been spoiled by its positioning by those who sell magical eating as merely a means to an end, that end being an altered physique. But being in our bodies and moving in ways that are pleasurable and sustainable are natural extensions of our humanness. Babies and children who have not yet become self-conscious about their bodies exude the joy they find in inhabiting them. It's a shame so many of us stop dancing, doing sports, or simply playing because we feel awkward, not good enough, or think that growing up means being in your head more than in your body. I am a huge proponent of doing things you are not good at simply because it feels good to do them. This is why I have taken up dancing with my toddler in our living room, long after stopping as a teen because I wasn't good at it and felt awkward in my body. Now the joy I get from grooving with my completely unselfconscious son is so much greater than any embarrassment I feel about dancing like Elaine on *Seinfeld*. For our current playlist, visit https://eat2love.com/eat-2-love-itunes-song-list.

Rediscovering embodied movement happens at its own pace. Begin to invite the pleasure of being in your body by bringing awareness to it as you go through the motions of your day. The core practice here is noticing. Noticing what it feels like to be in your body as you get out of bed, shower, and get ready in the morning, as you commute to work, and move about your normal routine. Meditation supports this practice of noticing; we sit and place our mind's attention on the feeling of the breath, and any time that strays we gently bring it back. Similarly, when experimenting with embodied movement, place your mind's attention on the feeling of being in your body. Whenever you find that attention has strayed, gently bring it back. Dropping into the body and holding your attention there familiarizes you with what it feels like to be embodied. As you become more familiar with this, try experimenting with moving your body in ways that feel playful, fun, and sensual. Walking, dancing, swimming, or trying a tango or belly dancing class are ways to reconnect with the pleasure of embodied movement.

Embodied movement also affects how our bodies relate to others. Caressing a beloved pet or, if you don't have one, volunteering at an animal shelter. Shaking hands with a new acquaintance, hugging and kissing your loved ones, and engaging in the most intimate activities. These are all examples of embodied movement. Holding hands in the movies, cuddling on the couch, masturbating, or making love: sexuality is a form of embodied movement that is part of who we are, yet many of us deny it or delay it due to fear and shame about our bodies. It takes courage and vulnerability to be in our bodies unselfconsciously when we get so many messages about how they aren't good enough as they are. The denial of our sensual and sexual selves is an unfortunate side effect of both the diet culture and the puritanical fear of pleasure. Reclaiming this fundamental aspect of ourselves is a vital form of ordinary generosity.

What types of physical discomfort have you been tolerating? Why do you deserve physical comfort and pleasure? How can you begin to bring more physical comfort and pleasure into your life?

What does embodied movement mean to you? How could you begin to bring more embodied movement into your life?

2. The Generosity of Fearlessness

In spite of the omnipresence of magical eating, some little voice inside is telling you to seek another way. And if history is the best predictor of the future, which likely means that diet after diet (or lifestyle change after lifestyle change) will continue to fail you and only lead to more suffering, choosing a different path and fully committing to it is the only sane response. This is a truly fearless act.

You weren't born thinking that food was dangerous and your body was wrong. Quite the contrary. You were programmed to think these things because the culture we live in values thinness over wellness. Skinny over sane. Clean eating over compassionate living. It makes you feel crazy. Fearlessness is the ability to see through your programming. Dr. Gail Dines, an anti-pornography activist, writer, and professor, has famously said, "If tomorrow, women woke up and decided they really liked their bodies, just think how many industries would go out of business." Let that sink in for a moment. Think about all the businesses targeting women that exploit your desire to be thinner, fitter, sexier, younger looking, different.

With the generosity of fearlessness, we begin to directly and indirectly disrupt the magical eating culture. By doing this, we reinforce that we are in charge of our bodies and communicate to others that a different world exists beyond our conditioning. The three forms of fearlessness are: (1) how you care for your body, (2) how you present your body to the outside world, and (3) how you talk about your own and others' bodies.

Caring for Your Body

We have already touched on the importance of eating satisfyingly throughout the day and giving yourself absolute permission to eat what, when, and how much you need to feel you have enough. We also discussed the generosity in allowing yourself to feel comfort and physical pleasure from non-food-related sources. With the generosity of fearlessness, we take caring for ourselves even further. Depending on access, this includes regular and preventive medical care. Scheduling those primary care, gynecologist, ophthalmologist, audiologist, podiatrist, dermatologist, and dentist appointments you have been putting off. (Including seeing your gastroenterologist for a colonoscopy. I never promised this was all going to be fun.) It means establishing boundaries in terms of how we spend our time, how we spend our money, how we let people treat us and speak to us. It means putting yourself first, especially if you have a habit of prioritizing others. It means saying "no" if your volunteering hand is normally the first to shoot up in the air so that you are not spread so thin you don't take care of your own body, mind, and heart. It means continually coming back and asking yourself if you are getting the basics of eating consistently and satisfyingly, drinking enough water, getting enough sleep, doing things that you enjoy, experiencing pleasure and sensuality, and spending time with people who lift you up.

Perhaps the most fearlessly generous thing we do in caring for our bodies is to allow ourselves to feel the full range of emotions, including difficult ones like fear, anger, sadness, shame, loneliness, boredom, and uncertainty. Explore them further by journaling, talking with friends, or speaking to a counselor or therapist. As a result, you may find yourself working with these strong emotions for the first time and being more authentically who you really are, or perhaps asking for help or support from a dietitian, therapist, counselor, or coach.

What are some fearless actions you could take to care for your body, mind, and heart? What might get in the way of caring for yourself in this way? How can you begin to work with this conflict to treat yourself with fearless generosity?

Presenting Your Body to the Outside World

This second form of fearlessness reinforces your Eat to Love path and communicates to others how you feel about yourself. This includes the posture you assume, how you dress yourself, and the activities you participate in. Rather than trying to make yourself as small as possible, begin to fully occupy the physical space your body needs. When standing, sitting, in a group and alone, at work and at home, on subways and planes, in restaurants and waiting rooms, in your clothes and in the shower. Take up the space you require. With this form of fearlessness, you might begin to do some of the things you have avoided or delayed because of your body. Confidently pose for a picture or put on a bathing suit and go swimming. Wear a sleeveless top, crop top, shorts, or horizontal stripes. Perhaps this is when you discover, or rediscover, your true personal style instead of choosing clothing others deem flattering or that camouflage your "problem areas." You might get off the sidelines and dance as you have longed to or set up an online profile and go out on some dates. Maybe you start having the sex you have always wanted to with your long-term partner or someone new (or yourself). When you renounce hating your body, you might reconnect with your sexual and sensual being, recognizing how healing and integrating this is. Even sitting down and meditating is a fearless act of being with your mind and body as they are, one that helps you to organically know who you truly are.

How can you change the way you occupy space? Play with your personal style? Reconnect with your sensual and sexual self?

How You Talk about Your Body and Other Bodies

This is the third form of fearlessness. There is a certain accepted language many of us use when speaking with others that is as predictable as reading a script. Fat talk, diet comparisons, and body bashing, of ourselves or others, are ways of bonding and finding common ground, particularly among women. The path of fearlessness includes disrupting this conditioned language and having new conversations. The simplest way to disrupt such talk is to not participate, to stonewall, to walk away, or to stand in silence while others wonder why you are not engaging. This interrupts the momentum of such exchanges and offers you or anyone else who wants to talk about more enlightening subjects a chance to introduce another topic. Refraining in this way requires great bravery. When you first try, expect to feel a certain amount of anxiety, which will naturally rise, level off, and then dissipate as you sit with it, again something your meditation practice trains you to accommodate.

A more direct approach to disrupting these conversations includes calling out biased talk and making the connection between it, weight stigma, and fat bias in our culture. Even if you do find yourself participating in this type of dialogue, it is important not to beat yourself up. Changing neural pathways is hard work (more on this in the chapter on the paramita of discipline). Noticing, reflecting, becoming nonjudgmentally curious, and resolving not to get hooked next time is a fearlessly generous way to respond. These actions free you and others up to have deeper, more meaningful conversations about things that matter.

How can you disrupt the conditioned language of magical eating? When confronted with others engaging in diet talk, fat talk, and body bashing, how could you respond? What do you observe when you disrupt the language of magical eating?

3. The Generosity of Sharing the Dharma

With the third form of generosity, we share the dharma. In this case, the dharma is the truth about what magical eating and self-aggression have cost us personally and as a society. We share this with ourselves and with others to open their eyes to a new way of relating to themselves and their world. This in turn reinforces our commitment to treating ourselves with generosity and crystallizes the insight gained from doing so.

Fighting against our bodies does not work and is in no one's best interest. To skillfully share the dharma with others, first consider what magical eating has cost you in terms of mental and physical energy, emotional pain, money, time, and lost enjoyment or experience.

Which of the following costs of magical eating have you experienced?

Mental and physical energy:

- Worries about your body shape or size
- Imagining that others are noticing or judging your eating, your body, and your character
- Learning the rules of various diets and trying to follow them
- Mentally categorizing foods as good and bad according to a revolving door of different diets
- Obsessing over foods you really want but won't allow yourself
- Anxiety that you might be eating the wrong foods
- Fear that eating certain foods is secretly affecting your body, brain, and health in negative ways
- Guilt for indulging in foods you've labeled as bad
- Anxiety about eating too much
- Fear of weight gain
- The emotional roller coaster of weighing yourself
- Feeling remorseful and physically uncomfortable after overeating
- Eating to avoid feeling uncomfortable emotions that probably needed to be experienced

- Feeling out of control with food
- Fantasizing about how life would be different if you were thinner, more together, less emotional, and basically a different person
- Loss of the fleeting elation when thinking about or starting a new diet or cleanse
- Feeling confused and disappointed when another diet fails
- Comparing yourself with others (including yourself ten years ago) and despairing at how you don't measure up

Money spent on:

- Maintaining a wardrobe in three different sizes
- Diet foods modified to be lower in fat, carbs, sugar, gluten, etc.
- Juice cleanses
- Protein powders and smoothie mixes
- Overpriced blenders
- Diet food delivery services
- Dieting books
- Dieting apps
- Diet service memberships
- Supplements or special foods to reduce appetite or speed up metabolism
- Unused exercise DVDs
- Unused gym memberships
- Unused exercise classes
- Unused exercise equipment, abdominal toners, etc.

Time expended on:

- Combing websites and forums for diet tricks, tips, and recipes
- Scrolling through Facebook, Twitter, Instagram, and Pinterest for diet tips, success stories, and before-and-after pics
- Fretting over what to eat, when to eat it, and whether it's good or bad
- Talking about your diet, food, weight lost, and weight gained instead of more interesting topics

- Doing exercise you don't enjoy in order to earn your calories or do penance for food already eaten
- Hovering too long over a menu deciding what's safe to order while everyone waits
- Lingering in supermarket aisles determining which foods to allow yourself and which to avoid
- Planning and executing a binge when restricting becomes too much to take
- Obsessing over what you just ate and feeling terrible about yourself
- Staring at your image in the mirror and dissecting your body with a mental Sharpie into the parts that are acceptable and the parts that must change

Enjoyment or experience lost:

- Avoiding certain eating environments such as public restaurants or going out to eat with friends for fear of judgment or of not being able to stay on a diet
- Opting out of activities with friends and families for fear of judgment about your body, fitness level, or eating
- Withdrawing from relationships, whether romantic, sexual, friendship, work, or casual, because of shame and fear of judgment about your body
- Avoiding favorite foods, or never discovering what those really are, because they weren't allowed on your diet
- Missing out on the types of movement and activities you enjoy because you chose exercise based on number of calories burned and never figured out what you really like
- Missing out on being silly and having fun in public for fear of drawing attention to yourself
- Missed opportunities to go out on dates, dance in public or private, and have intimate, sexual, and sensual relationships with others (or even yourself)
- Failing to learn how to deal with difficult emotions like sadness, loneliness, anger, fear, and restlessness without emotionally overeating

- Postponing trips to the places you want to visit, trying new activities, taking classes, and other things you have always wanted to do until you've lost weight, or perhaps not even knowing what those things are
- Missed opportunities to see yourself as anything but beautiful, desirable, and inherently lovable

Admitting what magical eating has cost us is startling. It is natural to feel anger at the culture that has oppressed us, sadness at what we have lost, and frustration and hopelessness that we still feel somewhat caught up in this damaging cycle. As we allow ourselves to feel the full weight of what magical eating has taken from us, we might also grieve the loss of diets and the structure and hope they provided and fear the uncertainty and groundlessness of a future without them. Anything you feel right now is completely okay, perfect even, and completely compatible with moving forward and learning a new way of taking care of yourself.

Magical eating with the goal of changing our bodies is a waste of our precious and limited time, energy, money, and experience. Not only does it not work, it also makes us feel terrible about ourselves. When we place a disproportionate amount of value on how much we weigh or on the potential dangers of what we eat, we lose focus on the other aspects of ourselves. We find it more difficult to appreciate the various and wonderful qualities that make us human. We disconnect from our core values and spiritual selves.

Magical eating also contributes to the development of eating disorders such as anorexia, bulimia, binge eating disorder, orthorexia, or an obsession with food, eating, and exercise. Even if not taken to such extremes, magical eating traps us in cycles of gray-area disordered eating that never raise red flags to get the attention, support, and healing required. And, like any addictive behavior, it makes us isolate, withdraw, and turn inward, essentially taking us away from life, from engaging with others, and from being in the moment.

Understanding what magical eating has cost you also expands your awareness of how much other people have been affected, how they too suffer with self-aggression, a lack of self-confidence and trust, pain and confusion about eating in a disordered way, and fighting with their bodies. Recognizing this helps us generate great compassion for others and may lead us to insights into how to help ourselves and others.

Armed with the knowledge of the price magical eating exacts, we can share that awareness with others. Sharing the dharma regarding magical eating could comprise talking about your own experiences of using magical eating to create the illusion of safety and certainty. Share your knowledge of how diets ultimately lead to weight gain, how weight cycling is more dangerous than living in a bigger body, and how the binge-restrict cycle only leads to greater suffering and rarely weight loss. Or share your personal journey of eating according to internal sensations versus external cues, practicing meditation, and being more compassionate toward yourself and others. Some of the ways in which clients and I have role-played this include:

- "I'm taking a different approach in which my wellness and happiness are more important than my weight, and I've never felt better."
- "Did you know that dieting is the best predictor of weight gain? I've given up dieting and am learning to listen to my body."
- "Have you ever wondered what it would be like to just stop hating our bodies and fighting against them? Dieting has never done anything good for me so I'm trying something different."
- "I've realized that talking like this only makes me feel worse about myself and my body. I'm just not doing it anymore."

How can you share the dharma of the Eat to Love path with others? What phrases might you keep in mind?

One of the simplest ways of sharing the dharma includes asking others to support you on your Eat to Love path. In the past, perhaps you enlisted the watchful eye and "helpful" advice of friends and family members to police you when you faced temptation, cheated, or wanted to give up on a diet that was causing you grief. Now that you are taking a different approach to eating and treating your body with generosity and compassion, sharing the dharma means letting them know those particular services are no longer needed. Even if confused at times, our loved ones usually only want what is best for us. Because they too are ensnared in magical eating, they do not see what that is. Whether because we used to ask them for one kind of support and now need a totally different kind, or because they face their own eating and body-related challenges and confusion, friends and family need specific guidance on how best to support you. Clients and I role-play these types of exchanges as well.

In response to others commenting about food:

- "I'm learning to listen to my body to tell me what, when, and how much to eat. It would be so helpful to me if you would trust that my body knows what's best and not comment on my choices."
- "I'm learning that there's no such thing as good and bad foods and that thinking about food in that way only contributes to harmful black-and-white thinking and behavior. When we're together, would you please not talk about food and eating that way?"

In response to others commenting on your body or weight:

- "I understand that you're trying to be helpful but your comments about my body really hurt my feelings. I'm learning to treat my body with kindness, generosity, and compassion and it would be so helpful to me if you would do the same. Do you think you could support me in this way?"
- "I'm taking a different approach that places my wellness and happiness above the number on the scale. It feels really great to treat myself in this way but it's a big change and not always easy. Do you think you could support me by not making comments about my weight or my body?"

To share the dharma with medical professionals, see my guide on how to navigate a Health at Every Size–ignorant healthcare system and download the free information card to share with your provider at https://eat2love.com/2017/12/01/navigating-haes-ignorant-health-care-system.

How can you ask others to support you on your Eat to Love path? What phrases might you keep in mind?

Other ways to share the dharma include changing what you consciously (and unconsciously) consume, which has a direct impact on what stories the media covers, what images companies promote, and what messages are considered culturally acceptable. From magazines and books to social media platforms, radio shows, and podcasts, immerse yourself in those that align with the Eat to Love path. Detox your bookshelf or Kindle of all diet books, including those masquerading as health resources (for instructions on how to permanently delete these books from your Kindle, see https://eat2love.com/2017/12/15/end-year-cleansefor-kindle); unfollow all diet, health, thinspiration, fitspiration, and before-after podcasts and social media feeds on Facebook, Twitter, Instagram, and Pinterest; cancel health magazine subscriptions that promote magical eating in any form; and patronize fitness experts who do not pit calories in against calories out for weight-loss purposes. Instead, inspire yourself to engage fully with your life by surrounding yourself with images of thriving people who look like you (and different from you). Immerse yourself in resources that emphasize eating and moving to feel well and accepting your body and treating it with kindness and respect, by supporting brands, organizations, and companies that do not discriminate against people of size (or on any other basis), and by contributing to the creation of a world in which all bodies are treated with equality, dignity, and compassion. Some compatible resources to immerse yourself in this path can be found in appendix D.

How can you change what you consciously and unconsciously consume in terms of traditional media, social media, and beyond?

Even if you choose never to utter a word about being on the Eat to Love path, the transformation that takes place in you will be noticed by others and could plant a seed that ripens in the unknown future. You will be modeling for others how you accept yourself right now and still continue to improve your relationship with food and your body. Giving to others in this way is self-perpetuating and sustains the ability to be generous to yourself.

Practicing generosity on your Eat to Love path is a fiercely courageous thing. Because this approach is still somewhat counterculture, you may feel like a salmon swimming upstream. Taking the risk of interrupting the momentum of magical eating conversations, putting yourself and your new journey out there for others to see, and generally upsetting the culture by stepping out of the shadows and no longer delaying your real life may make you feel vulnerable and raw. At the same time, you might begin to see glimpses of what it is like to live your life by trusting your body and yourself. Any time you feel exhausted from stretching into unfamiliar territory, you must come back down and rest.

Rest in the nature of alaya, the essence

This lojong slogan reminds us that there is something to trust and some place to come back to on this twisty turny path: the natural spaciousness of your own mind. *Alaya* translates as the essence, who we really are. As we touched on earlier in this chapter, there exists in your mind a pure awareness that is pre-concept and pre-judgment, something that cannot be encapsulated by even the most rudimentary terms of positive, negative, or neutral. This is who you are. The essence of humanness and the essence of basic goodness. This is the space to come back to any time you feel overwhelmed, alone, unsure, or exhausted. In those moments, you could say to yourself, "In this moment, I feel _____. It won't last forever but right now I need to come back to the simple spaciousness of my own mind and rest." Your meditation practice is the strongest invitation for the spaciousness of alaya, both on and off the cushion. In your meditation practice, there is nowhere to go. There is nothing to do but to feel your body breathing. This space is always there for you and, even if not initially, your practice will begin to feel like home: a place to rest.

Practicing the paramita of generosity is the most powerful beginning (and middle, and ending) to being on the Eat to Love path. Using the tools of connecting with the raw, unadulterated brilliance of your senses, continually coming back to your basically good and intelligent body, and bringing ordinary generosity, fearlessness, and sharing the dharma, all built on the foundation of your meditation practice, creates a strong basis for meeting your body where it is and taking good care of it.

THE PARAMITA

OF DISCIPLINE

IETERS ARE NO strangers to the word discipline. Discipline in Western society is associated with restraint, following laws, and punishment. For many of us, the word discipline means observing strict rules, always being "good," resisting temptation, and sticking to grueling workout regimens. Maybe discipline was what told you to track the time, type, and carefully measured amount of food you ate. To decline some tasty but potentially fattening morsel, thinking to yourself, *A moment on the lips, a lifetime on the hips* (how I hate that one). Perhaps discipline felt like a friend when it woke you up at dawn for another sweaty workout that you only enjoyed once it was over (instead of something you actually looked forward to).

A common definition of discipline is "the practice of training people to obey rules or a code of behavior, using punishment to correct disobedience." Outside of the military, boarding school, or jail, I can't imagine an environment where this feels more true than in magical eating, where there is a clear code to obey and penance (usually self-imposed) for any infractions. The problem with this when applied to eating and our bodies is that it backfires. Such rigidity about what we should and shouldn't eat, even if we comply for a little while, rouses the rebellious dragon in each of us. Once that dragon has been awakened, it is difficult to lull him back to sleep. I happen to think that this is a good and completely natural thing. Eating is one of the first ways we establish our agency, autonomy, and separateness from our mothers. It remains a means of expressing our power throughout our lives. When that power is taken away from us, even if we willingly hand it over to someone we think knows better than us, there is a disconnect. Magical eating gaslights us and then we end up gaslighting ourselves (and unconsciously participating in the gaslighting of others), all of which causes us to lose trust and self-confidence.

Sometimes we react to this conflict and confusion by becoming even more disciplined. But eventually the figurative pendulum swings in the opposite direction, and instead of ignoring our physical hunger and fullness sensations by undereating, we ignore and override them by overeating. Either way, we are not responding to our body's actual needs. By the time we have decided that this approach to discipline isn't working and that we wish to take back control over our bodies, we doubt ourselves, question our judgment, and have become numb to the internal sensations telling us what, when, and how much to eat.

Fortunately for us, the Buddhist meaning of discipline is very different from the militant one. It has nothing to do with harsh codes of conduct or penalties for misbehavior. Instead it is about coming back to our bodies, which are always in the present moment, again and again. As Chögyam Trungpa Rinpoche said, "Discipline is about giving up the search for entertainment." It is being with what is, right now, with gentleness, precision, and even joy. Referencing our bodies as the primary and most important source of information about what we need, be it food or some other form of care, is the touchstone we return to with trust and relief. Our meditation practice supports the practice of discipline naturally and organically because it requires the same coming back; we place our attention on the feeling of the breath and whenever we realize we have become absorbed in thought, we let it go with precision and gently bring awareness back to the breath. This reinforces the habit of always coming back to our experience, the one true thing, which is always happening *now*.

Another way of thinking about discipline is the ability to discern or have discriminating awareness. Similar to shifting our allegiance from external signals to internal sensations of how to eat, having the ability to discern what is actually happening in any given moment and what our true needs are requires the practice of discipline. When working with generosity, we practice listening and responding to the information communicated by our intelligent bodies in terms of physical hunger and fullness. Using our ability to clearly recognize what our bodies are communicating allows us to respond in a pure and authentic way. We develop the capacity to recognize and respond to the physical sensations of hunger and fullness and we also develop the awareness of when they are absent.

Having an urge to eat when you are not physically hungry is not a problem. Again, Eat to Love is not the eat-only-when-you're-hungry diet. The choice to eat is always yours, judgment-free. At the same time, not being able to tell the difference between physical hunger and a hunger that is more emotional in nature could be problematic. Habitually eating when you are not physically hungry often means that deeper emotional needs are not being met. Even once we recognize the difference between physical hunger and emotional hunger but can only respond to emotional hunger by eating, we find ourselves in the double bind of neither meeting our actual needs nor developing more beneficial coping skills. This shatters self-esteem, shakes confidence, and threatens self-trust. The urge to eat emotionally is not something to shy away from or fear; it has something important to teach us.

Pediatrician and *Mindful Eating* author Dr. Jan Chozen Bays identified one of several kinds of hunger we all experience as "heart hunger." I've always been fascinated by the concept of a hungry heart. It beautifully captures that feeling of emptiness, a void that needs to be filled. When clients eat to feed the emotional hunger of their hearts and inevitably find themselves dissatisfied, I visualize the food going into their mouths, being swallowed, traveling down the esophagus, and arriving in their stomachs, coming so close but nevertheless bypassing its target, the heart. Eating to fill the void of heart hunger is never truly satisfying. Even though its original motivation is feeling better, any comfort that is gained is at best short-lived. Only with the discipline of first recognizing heart hunger and discerning what you actually need in those moments may it truly be soothed.

PAULA AND I had been working together for a few months when her husband suffered a minor stroke. Though Paula's husband was steadily recovering, it had been stressful for her to care for him in addition to her demanding job and also caring for her aging mother. It was at this point in our work together that we began focusing more on Paula's emotional overeating, particularly in the evenings.

Paula had already given herself absolute permission to eat what, when, and how much she wanted. At the same time, she sensed that there was more to her nighttime eating than simply craving certain foods and allowing herself to eat them. Before her husband's stroke, evenings were when the two spent quality time together, attending social events, cooking at home, or just cuddling on the couch. It was also when they were most likely to have sex, an important part of their relationship that changed abruptly when her husband got sick. Since the stroke, Paula's husband was also dealing with depression and often took to the couch alone in the evenings to zone out in front of the TV. One day, Paula walked into my office with a sad grin. She shared that she had had an epiphany the night before. After a physically satisfying dinner with her husband, Paula's husband again took to the couch while Paula retreated to the bedroom with an ice cream cone. Using the mindful eating techniques of attention and connection with the senses, she was proceeding to eat the ice cream cone slowly and sensually by herself when she started to cry. Paula realized that she missed physical intimacy with her husband and was trying to fill that void with food. Once she realized this, Paula could allow herself to feel the sadness and loneliness she had resisted and to acknowledge her own grief and loss. She decided to speak to her husband about entering counseling, both alone and as a couple, to deal with what they were experiencing separately and also find ways to maintain physical intimacy in their relationship as their bodies continued to change.

The paramita of discipline provides us with the tools we need to recognize when we are at the mental fork in the road, the transformation point at which we have a choice to go down a habitual pathway or to try something different. Research has shown that the brain is malleable and can be guided toward ways of thinking that align with wellness, compassion, and self-care. As I've said before, the mind is a much better target for our self-evolving efforts (when done with gentleness, of course) while the body remains something largely out of our control.

Neuroplasticity is the term that has been developed to describe the brain's ability to form and reorganize connections between cells in response to learning or different experiences. What does this mean for us? That it is possible to change our minds and teach an old dog new tricks. It's the *how* that makes this possible. I like to describe neuroplasticity in terms of hiking. When we're out on a trail, there's usually one clear path that has been blazed and then worn down by those who have traveled it time and time again. As we hike that main trail, we might notice a minor path off the main trail. Fewer people have taken that one but it exists nonetheless, and someone out there traveled it for the first time. The difference between the main trail and that side path is how many times they have been traveled. Habitual thoughts are like that main trail. Every time we follow the thread of a habitual thought, we reinforce its importance and perceived truth. If we identify a different way of thinking that would actually be more beneficial, we could choose to take the equivalent of that side path. Once is not enough to make that side path as accessible as the main one. We must travel that new path over and over again in order to make it more habitual.

Before we change deeply worn habitual thought pathways, we must recognize that we are at a transformation point. This means moving beyond being on autopilot, continually coming back to our bodies, and recognizing when we have arrived at a point at which we can either follow that familiar habitual path or try something new. Each time we come to a similar juncture, we are faced with that decision again. Reinforcing a new thought pattern or behavior requires the discipline of coming back as well as continued practice and gentleness, all of which are supported by our meditation practice.

Neuroplasticity figures prominently in the paramita of discipline, particularly regarding the ways we misuse food when working with heart hunger. When I first read the next lojong slogan, I began to see the overlap between the Buddhist teachings and our relationship with food and our bodies. It is essentially the origin of the idea for Eat to Love. Learning about this slogan, I realized that this single teaching was at the center of so much that we struggle with, not just with food and body image but with life in general. It captures our preference for pleasure and the lengths to which we will go to avoid pain. It says everything about our ability to see ourselves clearly and to work with our habitual tendencies to liberate ourselves from their grasp.

Three objects, three poisons, and three seeds of virtue

Contemplating this lojong slogan helps us to see our natural preference for pleasure over pain, to see how we substitute food and habitual body thoughts to feed those preferences, and to see how we can liberate ourselves from this destructive trap. First, some definitions.

The three objects are:

1. things we like
2. things we don't like
3. things we don't care about or are afraid to look at

The three poisons are:

1. grasping after the things we like (also known as passion)
2. resisting or trying to change the things we don't like (also known as aggression)
3. turning a blind eye to the things we don't care about or are afraid to look at, in a slightly different way than aggression (also known as ignorance)

The three seeds of virtue are:

1. freedom from passion
2. freedom from aggression
3. freedom from ignorance

Next, let's take a deep look at how the three objects, three poisons, and three seeds of virtue relate to food and body criticism.

Food as the Three Poisons

The main ways in which we substitute food for our true needs are to hold onto pleasure, to resist discomfort or pain, and to numb out. We eat to grasp onto pleasure, or we have uncontrollable cravings for foods we believe will bring us pleasure; we eat in order to resist or change our experience of painful emotions; or we eat to numb out and not feel anything. Though the foods we are eating are not literally poisonous, this type of relationship with them could be; using food as one of the three poisons obstructs the recognition of what is actually happening and how to authentically respond.

Grasping

Whether we are eating a favorite food that no longer tastes so good as we become satisfied, or we have reached the point of comfortable fullness during a meal, eating to grasp onto pleasure is chasing pleasure that is dissolving or has already dissolved, and no longer responding to what our bodies are communicating. In working with grasping, we first must notice what is happening and that our actions conflict with that. By coming back to the sensations in the body, we gauge whether a food has begun to taste less fabulous as our taste buds habituate to it or feel as our stomach is about to move beyond comfortable fullness. This is also when it is helpful to remember that all things are impermanent; all urges, emotions, and phenomena arise, level off, and then dissolve. Eating experiences also follow this predictable life cycle. While it is sad when an enjoyable meal ends, continuing to eat *as if* we could recapture the pleasure we felt when we first began will always fall short, leaving us confused, disappointed, and possibly even physically uncomfortable.

Once we notice the conflict between our bodies and our minds, we see grasping more clearly. This is the transformation point. Experiment with pausing, interrupting the momentum of acting in conflict with your body's needs, reflecting on the disconnect, and reminding yourself that the food will be there when you want it again, whether that means when you are physically hungry in a little while or when you simply desire that food ten minutes from now. Because you have absolute permission to eat, it is never your last chance to eat this particular food. If, on the other hand, you recognize your grasping but are not able to stop, this too is progress.

Seeing where we are presents us with choices we don't have when we can't see where we are. Noticing this, being gentle with ourselves, and acknowledging that we are on our own path allows us to get there when we get there. By allowing ourselves to be exactly where we are and letting go of getting somewhere further down the line, we acknowledge that the path *is* the goal. Based on this perception, success comes solely from our awareness and willingness to stay with our true experience. (Note: the experience of grasping onto the pleasure of eating may seem like evidence of food, carb, or sugar addiction, but, again, the science does not bear this out. If there is any addiction, it is to the experience of pleasure gained in the act of eating, usually in order to avoid discomfort ... see the following.)

Aggression

When we eat to resist or change painful or uncomfortable emotions, we try to substitute the pleasure of eating for what we deem undesirable. We all have a natural preference for pleasure over pain. But in always moving away from emotional discomfort by eating, our suffering actually increases. Not only do we fail to develop and practice valuable skills to nurture, soothe, and care for ourselves, we never learn what the difficult emotions have to teach us. What's more, the habitual use of food to avoid emotional pain may cause physical pain and illness, contribute to disordered eating and eating disorders, and alter our natural set point range (see page 30) because we are consistently eating more than our bodies truly need.

When we find ourselves eating to aggressively change emotional states, again we must begin by noticing that there is a disconnect between what our bodies are communicating and what we are acting out. Once we notice this, we find ourselves at a transformation point: we may choose to continue down the habitual path of eating to avoid discomfort, or try something new.

Ignorance

When we eat to numb out, perhaps bombarding our senses with simultaneous Netflix, social media, and Chunky Monkey ice cream, our goal is to feel everything—and therefore nothing. When we eat out of ignorance, one approach to returning to our true experience is to simplify. Ask yourself, *What can I do without in this moment?* If you are overwhelming your senses with various forms of entertainment, perhaps take away one of them. If you are overwhelming your senses with foods that are over-the-top spicy, textured, and flavored, consider focusing on just one at a time. Give something your full attention and see what arises.

In these moments, we turn toward what is happening under the surface, taking the risk to experience something profoundly uncomfortable with the hope of understanding ourselves better. We acknowledge with gentleness and compassion that we are in the unfamiliar territory of working with what is.

The Three Poisons Worksheet

THE FOLLOWING PROCESS can be used any time you notice yourself misusing food as one of the three poisons. Whether that means at home alone after a terrible day, standing in front of the refrigerator, or already elbow-deep in a bag of cookies, bring these steps to mind to contact the intelligence of your body and the insight of your heart.

When you experience an urge to eat (or have already begun eating) in the absence of physical hunger . . .

1. PAUSE and create space

Bring your awareness to your present-moment body
Take three deep, embodied breaths
Notice the sensations of breathing in your body in the moment

2. Ask yourself: *Am I physically hungry?*

Yes

No

Eat!

Go to #3

3. Ask yourself: *Which of the Three Poisons is the cause of me wanting to eat? (Go to next page)*

Grasping
amusement, pride, pleasure, love, contentment, relief, interest, joy, admiration, compassion

Aggression
sadness, guilt, regret, shame, fear, disappointment, anger, disgust, contempt, hate

Ignorance
boredom, numbness, feeling overwhelmed, disconnected from feeling

4. Once you have identified what you are feeling, drop the words and experience the feeling in your body

Where is it located?

Does it move?

Is it dense or light?

What color, shape, texture is it?

Does it come and go?

5. Now ask yourself: *What is my true need in this moment?*

Am I getting the basics: food, water, sleep, etc.?

Do I have sources of comfort, pleasure, intimacy, and soothing?

Do I feel ready for some private personal exploration?

Am I craving supportive attention from others?

6. Take the next right step for you.

By interrupting the momentum of habitual thoughts and actions, it is possible to identify exactly what we are experiencing. Pausing to breathe and to connect with our true needs gets us out of our heads and into our bodies (and hearts). To become more familiar and comfortable with the full range of our emotions, it is useful to characterize our urges as passion (grasping), aggression (resisting), or ignorance (numbing out) and describe what we are feeling as specifically as possible—using the cues in the worksheet (which are based on the Geneva Emotion Wheel developed by the Swiss Center for Affective Sciences) to help identify them. We experience thousands of emotions every day but the most basic include those considered relatively positive (interest, amusement, pride, joy, pleasure, contentment, love, admiration, relief, compassion), those considered relatively negative (sadness, guilt, regret, shame, disappointment, fear, disgust, contempt, hate, anger), and the absence of or ignorance to emotion. Naming what you feel helps you acknowledge, or turn toward, what is going on inside your heart. If it feels within your reach, let go of the words themselves and simply feel the emotion in your body.

Once you have identified what you are feeling, you are at the transformation point. By recognizing where you are, you are more apt to detect and meet your actual needs precisely. Even if you are not able to exactly identify what you are feeling in those moments, bringing attention and curiosity to your discomfort, and recognizing that food will not satisfy this need, is a form of self-care that will eventually invite greater insight. As you do gain this insight into your true emotional needs, you begin to understand how they are most likely to be met. Do they fall into the general categories of meeting your basic needs, comfort and pleasure, private personal exploration, or supportive attention from others?

Getting the basics includes safety and security, warmth and protection, adequate rest and relaxation, eating and drinking consistently and satisfyingly throughout each day, and moving our bodies in ways that feel good. When we are missing any of these, we turn to misusing food as a poor substitute. Again this desire to eat for comfort is instinctual and inherently good; it's just not going to satisfy for long because it is imprecise and does not address the actual issue.

As I explained in the last chapter on non-food-related ways to be generous to ourselves, physical comfort, pleasure, and soothing help us feel cared for and connected with our bodies, other people, and the world around us. It means acknowledging our human need for intimate relationships, sensual touch, and experiences that fill our hearts.

Private personal exploration could include journaling, listening to relevant podcasts, or reading online or in books about whatever you are experiencing. It might also be a time to sit quietly with your experience without doing anything, to practice shamatha meditation, or directly contemplate what you are feeling in a meditative state. Spend this time being with the feelings you previously avoided by eating. Private personal exploration moves us toward deeper understanding and insight. We might also feel motivated and ready to seek outside support from others.

Supportive attention from others includes reaching out to a partner, friend, family member, counselor, therapist, clergyperson, meditation instructor, nutrition therapist, or other helping professional. Whether to vent, process, manage, or work through what we are experiencing, the supportive attention of others allows us to stop feeling the shame and isolation of our secrets, externalize what we fear is most unacceptable about us, discover we are not alone, and work toward peace.

When do you find yourself grasping after pleasure? Aggressively resisting discomfort? Numbing out in ignorance? What allows you to notice you are using food as one of the three poisons?

Our Bodies as the Three Poisons

Just as food may be misused as one of the three poisons, we occasionally treat our bodies in similarly distracting and destructive ways. We grasp on to what we like, aggressively resist or try to change what we don't, and numb out to what we don't care about. It might seem counterintuitive, but treating our bodies in such harsh ways can actually feel familiar and safe. When other aspects of our lives feel chaotic, turning our negativity toward our bodies feels like taking control. Our distaste for uncertainty or powerlessness may be so strong that we develop a preference for even a negative certainty, such as the idea that our bodies are unacceptable. Treating our bodies as one of the three poisons might be exacerbated when we are under a great deal of stress; though we come to believe it is our bodies that are causing us pain, upon further exploration, we are usually able to retrace our emotional steps to identify something else that felt disorienting or painful.

There are parts of our bodies we are attached to or believe must be a certain way to deserve love and acceptance (passion). There are the parts we hate and want to change to garner approval (aggression). Finally there are the parts we disregard or don't even think about (ignorance). Objectifying our bodies as one of the three poisons might cause us to downplay other aspects of our lives, to compare our bodies with others (real, imagined, or technologically altered), to "body check" by measuring and monitoring body parts, to avoid looking at ourselves in mirrors or other reflective surfaces, or simply to feel "fat," meaning devalued and disgusted. If we were to quantify the proportion of our worth derived from the appearance of our bodies on a pie chart, compared to other aspects of our lives, such as our relationships, work, and spirituality, would it occupy a disproportionately large slice?

The antidote to treating our bodies as one of the three poisons is to rebalance our perspective in two ways: by re-evaluating our bodies more holistically and by placing our bodies in the context of what we value. As explored in the lojong slogan about the preciousness of a human birth, our bodies are basically good. They deserve to be appreciated in their entirety and to be treated with kindness and compassion. In contemplating the basic goodness of the body, we acknowledge that there are parts of our bodies that are easier to accept, those that are more difficult, and those that we don't even think about. When we inhabit our bodies as the instruments that move us through the world rather than treat them as objects to be honed and perfected for the viewing pleasure of others, something shifts. With this perspective, we are more likely to appreciate and treat all the different parts of our bodies with respect.

The Self-Compassionate Body Scan

ONE OF THE best ways to rebalance our perspective on our basically good bodies is with a self-compassionate body scan.

Put on clothing that is loose, non-restrictive, and comfortable. Lie down on a supportive surface such as a bed or yoga mat. Begin by taking a few embodied breaths, focusing on the feeling of the breath entering and leaving the body. Then bring the following statements to mind as you move your attention from the bottom of your body to the top:

My body is doing its best.
My body does not want me to suffer.

Feet Soles, heels, toenails, and toes. Support and adaptation. Skin, tiny bones, and muscles working together to always find balance and move me forward. Bunions, hammertoes, blisters, warts. How often my feet go without appreciation; I ask so much of them.

Ankles Bones, ligaments, and skin. How they bend and adapt to different surfaces to accommodate my movements.

Shins and calves The texture of the skin and hair that cover them. Bones, ligaments, tendons, blood vessels. The muscles that carry me, that are criticized for being too big or too small.

Knees Bones, skin, tiny muscles, ligaments, and tendons. Constantly absorbing shock, being flexible. Accumulating wear and tear; communicating pain. How they adapt to so many changes.

Thighs Front and back. The longest bones and the biggest muscles in the body. Part of my body that does so much work. Where I store fat for my safety. Skin, hair, stubble, and cellulite. The texture of the skin, the stretch marks. Evidence of how my body adapts to everything I have thrown at it.

Hips and pelvis Skin, hair, bones, muscles, and fat. Protection. My center of gravity. My source of power. A source of vulnerability. The home of my sexuality. What allows me to give birth, create, and experience sexual pleasure.

Buttocks Skin, fat, muscle. How they cushion me, support me, and protect me.

Abdomen Skin, hair, muscle, organs, fat. Stretch marks and scars. Freckles. The container of so many internal organs I never think about. Stomach, intestines, kidneys, liver, pancreas, uterus, ovaries, bladder. The center of operations while growing a baby. The location of so much adaptation and accommodation. The focus of so much self-criticism. The center of nourishment and growth.

Torso and chest Skin, bones, muscles, ligaments, fat. Container of heart and lungs. Center of operations and caretaking for the body. Ribs that protect. Tiny muscles that stretch and support. Breasts that grow and change over time, that feed a baby, that are with me from the beginning of life.

Back Bones, skin, muscle, and fat. Freckles, skin tags, bacne. Spine, vertebrae, nerves. Sensory receiver, accommodator, shock absorber, workhorse, and pain meter.

Arms Upper arms, forearms, hands, fingers, nails. Skin, hair, fat, bones, ligaments, tendons. Biceps and triceps. The site of so much criticism. Shoulders, underarms, nerves, and muscles. How we connect with one another.

Neck Throat, voice, breath. Skin, bones, fat. Eating and swallowing. Constantly changing skin. Spine, turning, adapting.

Face Skin, oily, ashy, dry. Acne, scars. Bones, hair, fat, muscles. Eyes, nose, mouth, eyebrows, eyelashes, ears. Cheeks, chin, forehead. Center of connection, expression, and communication. Site of constant change and movement.

Head Hair, color, texture, thick or thin, skull. Center of protection, perception, learning, change, and connection. Home to the senses of sight, hearing, smell, and taste.

Close your body scan by taking a few embodied breaths, again focusing on the breath entering and leaving the body.

What are the parts of your body you like or believe must be a certain way to feel good about yourself? How can you speak compassionately to these body parts?

What are the parts of your body you dislike and want to change to feel good about yourself? How can you speak compassionately to these body parts?

What are the parts of your body you don't care about or rarely think about? How can you speak compassionately to these body parts?

Treating your body as an object to be changed, whether by exercising to fit into your jeans from college, positioning yourself in a chair so that you take up as little space as possible, or angling your phone to take a selfie in which you appear thinner, only makes your world smaller. Viewing your body as the instrument you inhabit while you live your life, such as by marching for a cause, embracing someone you love, standing in front of an audience to speak on an idea that is important to you, makes your world bigger. And better.

Once we have worked directly with the basic goodness of our bodies in their entirety, we widen our perspective to place our physical bodies in the context of other values. If we were to reflect wholeheartedly, there are usually many things that we hold more important and meaningful than the size and shape of our bodies. Relationships with family, friends, colleagues, pets, and our community. The work we do and how we contribute to the world, even if that is simply through our one-to-one interactions with colleagues, patrons, patients, students, strangers, or faceless customer service representatives on the phone. The ways in which we spend our time, meditating, making art, dancing or singing, being in nature, showing our affection, connecting with the most important people in our lives, making love, helping others. How we practice our spirituality, connect with one another, and make sense of the world as we try to live a good life. These are the things that seem to define our lives in the end.

How do you feel when you treat your body as an object? How do you feel when you treat your body as an instrument? What do you value about your relationships, work, spirituality, and how you spend your time?

When we are stressed, physically or emotionally, it may be more difficult to access these new ways of thinking and behaving. For this reason, we should be very compassionate and patient with ourselves when we feel we are falling short. (More on this in the next chapter on the paramita of patience.) As the saying goes, "Old habits die hard," and this is in large part because stress often reverts us back to old patterns. The more we are able to rebound from and let go of those experiences and come back to our bodies in the present moment, the more likely we are to move in the desired direction in the long run. And the long run is what we are concerned with.

When you are fortunate enough to experience times of less stress, use them to your advantage, experimenting with this new way of working with your mind and shifting it toward healthier, more self-compassionate thoughts and behaviors. Just as our meditation practice reinforces the practice of coming back to the breath, the paramita of discipline supports coming back to the body over and over again to decipher what we are feeling and what we need. It is with this pure awareness that we are able to take the best care of ourselves.

THE PARAMITA

OF PATIENCE

T HE SUBTLETIES OF how we think about and care for our bodies are intensely private. Only we really see. From the first time it occurred to us as babies to assert our autonomy by saying "no" to another bite of mashed bananas to the first time we said "no" to a food for fear it would make us fat. From the moment we understood that our bodies allowed us to crawl and give us pleasure to the moment we realized certain parts of our bodies were wrong somehow. Every day we have tens of thousands of conscious and unconscious thoughts and judgments that reinforce how we feel about food, eating, and our bodies. The origins of these feelings go back so far it can be difficult to recall exactly when we started relating to food and our bodies in ways that were influenced by magical eating. By the time you are reading this, you have probably been marinating in magical eating and the thinking that your body needs to change for decades. All of that time means you should be very gentle with yourself in the process of shifting your allegiance from magical eating back to your internal wisdom. This brings us to the paramita of patience.

Patience is exactly what you would expect: giving ourselves time to adjust to a new way of relating to food, our bodies, and the world around us. With patience, we allow ourselves to unlearn harmful beliefs and habits and to learn (or remember) nourishing ones. We acknowledge that the duration and quality of this process depends

139

on our unique history and experiences. Patience teaches us to speak to ourselves with compassion and to forgive ourselves for the times when we are harmful or unkind to ourselves. Patience helps us to slow down our thinking about food, eating, and our bodies and to create space around the actions that we take. Rather than reacting out of irritation, frustration, or fear, we cultivate a new habit of non-reactivity. Having patience allows us to respond to new situations with gentleness and gives us the time we need to develop the unconditional trust that whatever obstacles arise are workable.

Cultivating patience on your Eat to Love path begins by recognizing the beliefs and behaviors that form your unique version of magical eating. Once you have acknowledged them, begin to contemplate them, question them, and poke some holes in their logic and validity. As you gradually break down the beliefs that tricked you into thinking you needed to change in order to be healthy, worthy, desirable, and happy, it is possible to replace those destructive beliefs with others that are in fact more true and based on your own personal exploration, experimentation, and communication with your intelligent body.

What are some of the key events that happened in your childhood, adolescence, and early and later adulthood that contributed to your unique magical eating and body thoughts? How many years have you carried these beliefs? What magical eating beliefs do you still hold based on these events?

Magical eating slowly solidified in your mind over the course of many years. Learning to trust your body and to use it as an instrument of your life, rather than treat it as an object to be chiseled to perfection, is an ongoing process that unfolds over a long and unknown course of time. Unlearning magical eating is not a fix-it-and-forget-it kind of deal. When clients come to me saying, "I just don't want to think about food anymore," I break it to them gently that they will always have to think about food (because everyone does!), but that they will think about it differently and in a way that is not distressing.

Many of us envision patience as grinning and bearing it or being existentially calm. Neither of these is necessary in order to practice true patience. Instead of gritting our teeth or white-knuckling it through the challenges inevitable on the Eat to Love path, we practice patience by letting go of expectations. We recognize what is arising in our bodies and hearts, turn toward it, and lean in. By doing this, we become familiar with what previously sent us running in the opposite direction. Rather than reacting immediately with passion, aggression, or ignorance, as we discussed in the last chapter on discipline, we respect whatever is happening with a willingness to feel it and to stay with it. As Sylvia Boorstein said in the name of one of her meditation books, *Don't just do something, sit there.*

Rather than acting out in habitual ways, our meditation practice supports us to be flexible and resilient in the face of discomfort and skillful in how we respond. We *choose* how to respond, that is, rather than acting on autopilot only to discover what happened later on (if at all). Practicing patience is inherently courageous. It strengthens our connection with our bodies, our minds, and our true experience.

Obviously, the notion of letting go of expectations runs wildly counter to magical eating, in which expectations rule supreme. Expectations of happiness, of problems suddenly disappearing, of finding love, of having hotter sex, of escaping suffering. Expectations are exactly what sell magical eating. And yet having such expectations, projecting into an imagined future about what might happen, takes us out of the present moment and disconnects us from what is actually happening in our bodies, hearts, and environment. Stripping away these expectations helps bring our attention and awareness back to our intelligent bodies. This change is often alien and very unfamiliar so the pace at which it unfolds must be respected.

BY THE TIME Adriana came to work with me she had been on one diet or another for more than thirty years. She had decided to never diet again and was very impatient to be healed from the damage done. As we began our work together, we both realized how strongly she held onto certain dieting beliefs, such as the importance of weighing herself and following a low-fat diet. With time, Adriana let go of these more and more. She threw out her scale, had assertive conversations with medical providers when she did not want to be weighed (because it wasn't medically necessary), and created and defended boundaries with family members. She let her tastes drive her eating and focused more on how her body felt as the result of the choices she made. She stopped drinking artificially sweetened beverages because she didn't really like the taste or how they made her stomach feel, and she discovered that her after-dinner sweet tooth was more of an occasional desire than a nightly one. She went through a period of intense anger about dieting and magical eating and how both had been foisted upon her by her parents, peers, and the culture. She was angry that she had delayed her life because she didn't have the "right" body. As she allowed herself to fully feel her anger, she moved through it and was eventually able to touch the deep sadness that was underneath. Adriana longed for more sensuality in her life. One belief that hung on from her dieting days was that she didn't deserve this until her body was smaller. Though she still faced challenges, she learned to speak to herself and her body as her dear friend would speak to her. As a result, she decided to take better care of herself and present herself to the outside world in a way that reflected that. She cut off her long hair, which was a radical act since she was always told that short hair was unflattering for her face shape, and started wearing dangly earrings. She started taking drumming lessons and salsa classes to bring more embodied movement into her life. One of my favorite things Adriana said during one of our sessions was "When did shame ever cause someone to heal?" We decided shame was more likely to make someone heel than heal.

Letting go of expectations and practicing patience means meeting ourselves where we are, wherever that may be. Each piece of the puzzle—physical hunger, emotional hunger, physical fullness, psychological fullness or satisfaction, embodied movement, and body image—exists on multiple levels. At the beginning, we have one understanding of how we have internalized magical eating. Only by recognizing and removing those first few layers of programming can we make way for the deeper understanding that comes as the result of staying on this path. Many clients have shared, with surprise, that even after years they discovered just how many dieting beliefs persisted in subtle ways. They couldn't appreciate these deeper beliefs until they were ready.

The greatest obstacle to patience is aggression: resisting whatever arises in our experience, acting out in habitual ways in order to change our experience, or wanting things to change faster than they naturally do. Look at the paramita of patience as simply allowing: allowing ourselves to be at the stage we are, allowing ourselves to experience the discomfort of unfamiliar situations and strong emotions, allowing ourselves to not know what the right answer is in certain situations, and allowing ourselves to make our best guess and continue to move forward.

Self-Compassion

The most useful tool in practicing the paramita of patience is self-compassion. Many of us have made the mistake of thinking, *If I'm hard on myself, I'll feel motivated and achieve my goals.* Several clients have pointed to all the ways in which being hard on themselves culminated in diplomas, promotions, publications, raises, and other achievements. And yet this approach always fails when it comes to the care and feeding of our bodies (and likely had consequences when applied to other situations as well). We might imagine that we will be kinder to our bodies when they change at some unknown point in the future, when we lose weight, eat clean, or look a certain way, but this is just another way in which we get it backward. If being so harsh with ourselves could ever motivate us to lose weight or take better care of ourselves, wouldn't it have worked by now? Acknowledging that it hasn't is a very good reason to consider the possibility that the path of harshness and self-aggression is fruitless when it comes to self-care and that gentleness is worth trying.

Learning new ways of caring for your body and working with your thoughts is challenging. When you have struggled with food and body as long as many of us have, there will inevitably be a period of unlearning some things and relearning others, of gradually trusting our bodies and our judgment again, and accepting the uncertainty inherent in not following prescriptive rules. For the changes going on in both our bodies and our minds, developing nonjudgmental curiosity and self-compassion is essential.

Kristin Neff, PhD, researcher and author of the book *Self-Compassion: The Proven Power of Being Kind to Yourself*, has identified the three central components of self-compassion as: treating ourselves with kindness rather than judgment when it comes to our mistakes, shortcomings, and imperfections; recognizing that everyone experiences suffering, imperfection, and vulnerability—we are not alone; and seeing negative emotions and experiences as they are, neither exaggerating nor downplaying them. Self-compassion is not self-pity, which causes us to disconnect from others and to withdraw into our own suffering. It is not self-indulgence, which causes us to take a lopsidedly positive view of ourselves and not see ourselves with nonjudgmental honesty. And it is not self-esteem, in which we must always be above average, in which we must see ourselves as better than others, and which is contingent on continued success. People who practice self-compassion are more resilient, have a more truthful perception of themselves, enjoy deeper and more nurturing relationships, and experience less narcissism and reactive anger. Compelling research also suggests that people who take a self-compassionate view of their bodies—that is, they are honest, nonjudgmental, and treat themselves with absolute respect and kindness—tend to take better care of themselves.

A first step toward becoming more self-compassionate is recognizing the ways in which we speak to ourselves. Many of us have internalized a voice that tells us when we have been good or bad. A voice that criticizes our bodies, shames us for eating certain foods, or berates us for not achieving an impossible ideal. This voice is like a soundtrack that plays non-stop in the back of our minds. Noticing that you have a tendency to speak to yourself with harshness is not another opportunity to be hard on yourself; most of us struggle with being hard on ourselves in some areas of our lives. The point of noticing is to generate awareness, become familiar with its nuances, and begin to work with our minds to become gentler and more compassionate.

TO THE OUTSIDE world, Chelsea was intelligent, witty, and dry. To herself, however, she was very harsh. Chelsea had learned from an early age that the worst thing a girl could ever be was "full of herself," so she learned to preemptively cut herself down to size. Though she was kind to others, she did not extend this kindness to herself in her internal soundtrack. Chelsea's harshness extended to all corners of how she related with herself. She fought with her hunger, denying it until the breaking point when she binged. She fought with her body in running because she wasn't the fastest. Before we started working together, Chelsea thought that being harsh with herself would motivate her to be better. It wasn't until she began to pay closer attention to her internal soundtrack that she realized how negative and critical it was; that it was not motivating her but rather causing her to hate herself. Because harshness felt second-nature and safe, Chelsea was skeptical of becoming self-compassionate. But she trusted the process and continued to come for weekly sessions to work through her negative thoughts, even though she would try her best to poke holes in my every argument about why she deserved compassion. Gradually, we discovered that Chelsea had begun relating to herself more frequently as good enough. She even had an experience where she saw her reflection in a mirror and judged herself positively before fully realizing it was her. Eventually Chelsea could be more compassionate, humorous, and not shaming toward herself, though she still phrased things in her own authentic snarky voice. "Hating yourself won't ever lead to self-improvement," she said in one of our last sessions together. I had to chuckle at that one.

What are the most frequent self-criticisms that are part of your personal soundtrack? Say them aloud one by one and feel what it's like to hear them this way, perhaps for the first time.

What thoughts and feelings wash over you when you hear these statements? Where do you feel it in your body? What does it feel like in your heart? Based on how each statement makes you feel, how has this affected how you approach eating, embodied movement, and self-care?

When you speak your personal soundtrack out loud, you might be surprised at just how malicious you are to yourself. Many of my clients have been struck by the viciousness of their words to themselves, remarking that they would never think of saying these things to their friends, children, sisters, or mothers. Now, with the awareness of how your soundtrack affects your self-care, could you imagine a state of mind in which you didn't feel this way? Could you imagine what it would feel like *not* to be so hard on yourself? What it would feel like to demote culturally established beauty ideals on your list of priorities? What do you feel when you glimpse, for just a moment, the absence of this self-criticism? Bring your awareness to this practice as often as you like, knowing that it can be difficult to connect with or maintain but that even in those flashes of clarity, there is space and possibility.

Once you have explored in some detail the very real effects of your personal soundtrack on how you feel and how you care for yourself, consider each statement again. See if each criticism could be reframed in neutral terms. For example, *My stomach rolls are disgusting* could become *This is a human stomach, it's white/pink/brown/black and soft and round.* Removing the judgment from our soundtrack and replacing harsh criticism with neutrality brings some space into our hearts and minds and helps us to see things as they are, neither inherently negative or positive.

How can you begin to reframe your soundtrack statements so that they become neutral statements?

With time and practice, neutral statements can again be reframed to be compassionate. *This is a human stomach* may eventually transform into *This is my stomach, it is so much more than rolls of fat. It houses my internal organs, runs on its own, and adapts to countless changes, including growing another human being. My stomach is a part of my body that deserves care and acceptance simply because it exists.*

How can you further reframe your neutral statements so that they become self-compassionate statements?

Having self-compassion does not mean never having a negative thought about your body. As much as we work toward cultivating absolute permission to eat, we have absolute permission to think. That means that no thought is forbidden; all are welcome. Meet negative or self-aggressive thoughts by turning toward them, by trying to discover where they come from, and by finding a way to respond to them on neutral terms and gradually with more warmth and compassion.

Just as we bring patience and self-compassion to our internal soundtrack, we bring them to the many obstacles we encounter on the Eat to Love path. Magical eating is all about avoiding mishaps: eating before you go food shopping, drinking a big glass of water before a holiday meal, hanging around the veggie platter at a cocktail party and not setting foot near the cheese board. But the Eat to

Love path welcomes mishaps. The more, the merrier. We don't aim to avoid obstacles, rather, we bring them along because they have much to teach us.

One of my favorite concepts in Buddhist philosophy is that everything you encounter should be brought to the path. Every thought, feeling, reaction, and interaction should be contemplated as part of understanding the nature of reality and indeed yourself. This seems especially true of the ways in which we relate to food and our bodies.

When the world is filled with evil,
transform all mishaps into the path of bodhi

In this lojong slogan, *evil* represents anything that distracts from or discourages your attention and allegiance to your body's intelligence. *Mishaps* are the obstacles that arise on this path; they may feel problematic but are nevertheless essential to a deep and true understanding of how to care for yourself. And the *path of bodhi* is this path of Eat to Love, which you travel as a bodhisattva, central to which are compassion and awareness of what is going on in your body and mind from moment to moment and a willingness to always come back to that with curiosity and without judgment.

Because the diet culture's magical eating reinforces dualistic thinking, in which foods are either good or bad and decisions right or wrong, it is easy to get knocked off balance. According to that narrow-minded approach, one misstep may mess the whole thing up. Many clients describe dieting experiences in which they make one choice, eating a cookie or a whole bag of cookies, that throws them off to the point that they stop bringing any attention to how they eat for the remainder of the day and vow to start over the next day with a clean slate.

On our path, there are no wrong decisions and no bad foods. We do not sustain such black-and-white thinking. The so-called mishaps on this path could be mistaken for evidence that it is not working for you. Instead these mishaps are opportunities to deepen your understanding of your body and your mind and to expand your tolerance for uncertainty and discomfort, both of which are essential to the care and feeding of yourself (and to your life in general). What follows are some of the most common mishaps or obstacles on the path to eating and treating our bodies compassionately. As you work with them, consider revisiting the Three Poisons Worksheet on page 128, which helps you identify and acknowledge exactly what you are feeling as well as how to move forward with gentleness.

Forgetting to Connect with the Senses

Just as we aim to inhabit our bodies by connecting with the senses when we eat (as well as when we aren't eating), we aim to notice when we are *not* in our bodies. Because of the different narratives about what we should and should not be eating and which foods contribute to health and which to weight gain or disease, it is not uncommon to be eating with our bodies while our minds are elsewhere. The most common obstacles to connecting with the senses include regular distraction, guilt/anxiety, and intentionally disconnecting from our current experience to change how we feel.

With regular distraction, we place our awareness on some form of entertainment while eating, so that we are not fully present. When we do this we are likely to miss the sensual aspects of the food and the satisfaction that comes from observing our physical and emotional responses to eating. Regular distraction may also cause us to eat more than we need to feel satisfied by missing the body's sensations of comfortable fullness. Choosing to eat mindlessly can be a part of a mindful eating practice, but the element of choice is critical. The antidote to regular distraction is to intentionally remove the things that absorb our attention or to focus solely on eating for a set amount of time. Take baby steps. Try eating the first bite of any meal with your full awareness. Next, try eating with full attention for the first five minutes of your meal. After the five minutes are over, give yourself permission to enjoy your favorite distraction. With time, you might discover that eating with attention is preferable to eating in a distracted way.

The second obstacle to connecting with the senses while eating is guilt or anxiety. Many of us lose our connection with our senses while eating because we feel guilt about eating something we think we shouldn't or anxiety about eating something we fear will lead to negative consequences, whether it be weight gain or ill health. When our bodies are eating and our minds are feeling guilty or anxious about it, we are much less likely to eat according to our internal sensations. We may eat more than we need to feel satisfied because we are secretly vowing *this is the last time*. Or we might cut short our meal, throw it in the garbage, and pour water on it to prevent us from eating any more. Either way, guilt and anxiety rob us of any joy from eating and prevent us from learning more about our true likes and dislikes. To feel guilty or anxious while eating would suggest that we have committed some sort of offense or have intentionally eaten poison, but how is this possible if all we are doing is consuming some chocolate cake or crunchy cheese doodles?

Feeling guilty and anxious about eating is a byproduct of magical eating that assigns a moral quality to food. This type of thinking is an emotional dead end; there is no way to work with it. Magical eating would have us reinforce dysfunctional thoughts and behaviors, leading to further suffering. The antidote to feeling guilty or anxious about eating is giving yourself absolute permission to eat, with the intention of connecting with your internal sensations and true experience: how your body feels while you are eating, an hour later, a day later. Often, when people let go of the anxiety about eating certain foods and really give themselves absolute permission, they don't have the expected reaction.

Even if you *are* eating a food that somehow doesn't work for you, whether because it upsets your stomach or gives you excessive gas (note: while it may not be enjoyable, a certain amount of gas is a normal part of having a body), feeling guilty or anxious still does not help. What does help is connecting with the body and acknowledging that while eating a certain food is enjoyable in the moment, it predictably leads to physical discomfort that you would prefer not to experience. Prioritizing not feeling physical discomfort over the enjoyment of eating certain foods occasionally gives rise to feelings of deprivation, sadness, or longing but need not be a problem. Absolute permission means you always have a choice in how to feed yourself and what to prioritize. (You will learn about this in greater detail in the chapter on wisdom.)

The third obstacle to connecting with the senses is when we intentionally disconnect from our bodies to change how we feel. Whether we are simply not acknowledging what we are eating, overeating emotionally, or in the midst of an all-out binge, our minds and our bodies are in very different places. By disconnecting with our bodies, we do not heed internal sensations, sense what is unfolding, or connect with what we really need. Some examples of this include overwhelming your senses with quantity or explosive sensual qualities as my client did with handfuls of peanut M&Ms, eating very quickly or expediting the time between the lips/teeth and swallow, and of course eating in an aggressive and punishing way that actually causes you to feel discomfort, illness, or pain.

The antidote to intentionally disconnecting with the body is more complicated than the other two. To begin to work with this obstacle, the core practice is noticing: noticing when there is a desire to disconnect and not feel or to feel something different. Often when we begin this form of noticing, we only become aware of what was going on after it has already happened. Think of this as *mindfulness after the fact* (but mindfulness nonetheless). With continued attention, practice, and gentleness, our mindfulness and awareness of what is unfolding moves closer and closer to real time. It may even progress to the point of anticipating what is about to happen because you have been down that road so many times and are familiar with how it unfolds.

The body is always with us. Our access to the senses is continuous. Yet despite the fact that we carry this wisdom with us at all times, we may forget to connect with the senses. As with any time we forget the basic instructions, the solution is to recognize we have forgotten, reconnect with them however possible, and resolve to do this again and again. This is as true for our Eat to Love practice as it is for our meditation practice. Even though I have been practicing meditation for about ten years, sometimes I forget the instructions. My technique gets too loose and I daydream more than meditate. When I realize this has happened, I seek out a reminder: reading about the meditation technique, listening to a guided practice, or even giving myself basic instruction. Similarly, once you realize you have forgotten to connect with the senses, consider coming back to the lojong slogan *Examine the nature of unborn awareness*, explained on page 77, or leading yourself through a mindful eating exercise, such as the one in appendix A.

Focusing on one sense at a time also heightens our awareness of and connection with the senses. Go outside into the world and contemplate your surroundings using primarily one sense at a time:

- Focus on your sense of sight in a garden, on a city street, at a museum, window shopping, or at a restaurant or shop you appreciate for its visual appeal and stimulation
- Focus on your sense of hearing at a beach, on a busy street, in a library, at a concert, listening to your favorite music
- Focus on your sense of smell in a flower shop, candle shop, bakery, pizza joint, or walking by a newly mown lawn
- Focus on your sense of taste with foods that hit the various taste buds of sweet, salty, spicy, sour, bitter, and umami
- Focus on your sense of different temperatures (hot, warm, cool, cold) and textures (crunchy or creamy, juicy or dry, crisp and raw, or cooked and soft)
- Focus on sensual touch with different textures, such as a silk scarf, running your hand across bricks or pavement, sand slipping through your fingers, water touching your skin, bare feet on the grass

When do you forget to connect with your senses while eating? How can you apply the antidote? How might you reframe the experience with compassion?

Getting Too Hungry / Not Eating Regularly

Our bodies need food and water at regular intervals throughout the day in order to function and thrive, yet we often fail to meet this need consistently.

CHLOE OFTEN ATE breakfast relatively early in the morning and then nothing until she came home from work late at night, when she overate comfort foods high in carbs and fat. She was barely conscious of hunger sensations that came and went throughout the day and found it easier to compartmentalize eating in this way so she was not distracted by such mundane details during her demanding day. As we worked to insert smaller meals or snacks at regular intervals, those natural hunger sensations gradually began to re-emerge. The more she responded to them, the more regularly they arose and the more familiar she grew to their nuances. Her evening binges also receded and she was able to make different food choices that aligned with varying tastes and satisfaction. Though she still struggles at times to feed herself consistently, Chloe realized that getting too hungry and not feeding herself regularly was the root of her problems.

When working with hunger and fullness, our goal is to avoid extremes. When we get so hungry that we cannot physically function, there is a natural tendency to eat in a way that sends us to the opposite extreme of feeling stuffed or even sick. Avoiding this extreme hunger by recognizing and responding to hunger signals when they are gentle but clear is the best way to avoid either extreme of famished or stuffed. Even if it is not always possible to feed ourselves a meal when we are hungry for one, stocking snacks in the office refrigerator, in a desk drawer, in the car, at home, in our gym bag, and in our purse helps us out in a pinch. Some ideas for satisfying and stockable snacks include:

- Homemade trail mix with nuts, dried fruit, and chocolate chips
- Energy bars with a good balance of protein, carbohydrates, and fat
- Whole milk yogurt with granola
- An apple or banana with nut butter

- Whole-grain crackers with nut butter and jam
- Hard-boiled eggs with carrots and hummus

Our choices don't have to be perfect. As long as we have the intention of listening to our bodies and doing our best to respond to them, we continue to confidently walk this path.

When do you find yourself getting too hungry? Why do you find it hard to feed yourself consistently? How can you work with this obstacle? How might you reframe this experience with compassion?

Bypassing Comfortable Fullness

Eating is a pleasurable experience and sometimes we experience real disappointment and sadness when that pleasure comes to an inevitable end. As you recognize and respond to comfortable fullness, wherever your middle way is, you might find yourself occasionally eating past this point. Bypassing comfortable fullness occurs for several reasons: rebelling against a long history of deprivation, subtle magical eating beliefs that include not giving yourself absolute permission, a desire to prolong the pleasure of eating, a resistance to the natural dissolution of an eating experience, and the avoidance of whatever it is we must return to once the meal has ended. It is our choice what level of fullness to eat to; there is no moral imperative to stop at your middle way. But if bypassing comfortable fullness has the unwanted effects of physical discomfort, ignoring concerns that would be better directly addressed, or just knowing that you can, it is worth taking a closer look.

One way of working with this dynamic is to stop at the moment you feel you have had enough, to mark it by putting down your fork and saying to yourself, silently or out loud (depending on the circumstances and social acceptability of talking to yourself), *I am pausing at this moment to feel what my body wants and needs.* Then, if you decide you wish to experiment with ending your meal at this point, continue with, *I give myself absolute permission to continue eating but I choose not to in this moment because* _____.

Fill in the blank with whatever feels true, whether it is *to discover what I really need in this moment, to appreciate the food I have just eaten,* or *to experiment with stopping before I am uncomfortably full.* Consider taking a ten-minute pause with the implicit understanding that you have absolute permission to continue eating at that point if you still would like to. During those ten minutes, you could write down what you experience, meditate, do ten minutes of whatever task you have been avoiding, or engage in some other activity that feels neutral or pleasurable.

When do you find yourself bypassing comfortable fullness? How can you work with this obstacle? How might you reframe this experience with compassion?

Mistaking Memory for Present-Moment Experience

Related to the obstacle of bypassing comfortable fullness, at times you might continue to eat past the point of enough because the food just tastes so good. When you connect with the senses and stay with your sense of taste throughout a meal, however, you might discover that it changes from one bite to the next. This is one of the first messages our body sends us to say it is becoming satisfied. When you eat as if the taste continues to be as vibrant as the first bite, it could be because you are actually holding onto the memory of that first bite rather than experiencing each subsequent one. Other times, a food does not even taste as good as you think it does because you are eating it while holding onto the memory of a previous time when it tasted better than now. The best and perhaps only way to work with this obstacle is to recognize that you are eating with your memory and not with your body and to bring your attention back to the actual experience as it unfolds.

DALE WAS ATTACHED to her two cups of morning coffee but found herself over-caffeinated much of the time. As we explored this, Dale shared how much she enjoyed the first half of her first cup of coffee when the temperature was just right, when the kids hadn't woken up yet, and when she had a few quiet moments to herself. But after that first half-cup, her enjoyment level decreased and her drive to drink coffee increased. Dale realized that the increased drive to drink her coffee even though she wasn't enjoying it was because of a desire to recapture the enjoyment of that first half-cup. Realizing this allowed Dale to let go of the second cup of coffee that didn't make her body feel good anyway and to really enjoy those first few perfect sips each morning, acknowledging the dissolution of the experience as it occurred.

When do you mistake memory for present-moment experience? How can you work with this obstacle? How might you reframe this experience with compassion?

Mistaking Quantity for Quality

Just as we sometimes confuse the memory of an enjoyable eating experience with an actual one, we might confuse quantity with quality.

JACKIE STOCKED AN ice cream that was a diet-friendly substitute for her favorite brand. But whenever it was in the house, she ate the whole container. Much of our first sessions together focused on this conundrum. What she realized, after working through this scenario over and over again, was that she was compensating for what she lost in the quality of the ice cream she really enjoyed—the full-fat, full-sugar version—with a greater quantity of the modified one. Once Jackie paid attention to the satisfaction (or lack thereof) from the diet ice cream and recognized that no quantity of it would ever feel like enough, she gave herself permission to eat her favorite ice cream and trusted her body to tell her when she had enough.

What Jackie experienced is not unusual—there's even a name for it: the Snackwell effect. People often eat more of a compromised version of a food to make up for the quality lost from eating the original. Recognizing this disconnect, reinforcing your absolute permission to eat, prioritizing satisfaction, and eating mindfully are how to work with this obstacle.

When do you mistake quantity for quality? How can you work with this obstacle? How might you reframe this experience with compassion?

Mistaking Stopping When Comfortably Full for Deprivation

Many clients have described experiencing resistance to stopping when comfortably full because it feels akin to deprivation. Deprivation they imposed on themselves over years of magical eating that they were now working to eradicate through giving themselves absolute permission. This obstacle contains within it information about whether you have fully or only partially given yourself permission to eat without restriction. If there is even the slightest doubt that you will be able to eat what, when, and how much you need to feel you have had enough, you might find yourself eating in this particular reactive way. The antidote to mistaking stopping when comfortably full for deprivation is again reinforcing the fact that you have absolute permission to eat and acknowledging with patience and self-compassion that you are still recovering from your history of deprivation. Eventually, the decision to stop eating is no more emotionally charged than the decision to continue.

When do you mistake stopping when comfortably full for deprivation? How can you work with this obstacle? How might you reframe this experience with compassion?

Eating Out of Boredom

Many people describe eating when they are not physically hungry, not out of a desire for a certain food but instead out of boredom. There are two kinds of boredom in Buddhist thought: hot boredom and cool boredom. Hot boredom feels like an allergic reaction to nothing happening. You might feel restless, twitchy, itchy, unable to sit still; it is a feeling of needing something but not being able to put your finger on it. Hot boredom is a reaction to the naturally arising spaces or gaps in our lives. The moments in which nothing in particular is going on. This freaks us the hell out. We live in a culture in which every moment is filled in with some form of entertainment, stimulation, and distraction. Noticing when our true experience is *nothing* is so unfamiliar that it feels uncomfortable, painful even, and in need of fixing. Hot boredom often sends people to the fridge, freezer, or pantry. The activity of picking up a piece of food, biting, chewing, swallowing, repeating again and again may feel preferable to the spaciousness of hot boredom. However, we miss something when we fill in every moment of space in our lives and habitually respond to hot boredom with eating (or any number of entertainments). Without allowing ourselves to feel hot boredom, we never move through it to feel cool boredom.

Cool boredom is what we are inviting when we sit down to meditate. We still our bodies, settle our minds, and see what arises without agenda. That often reveals how we will stop at nothing to entertain ourselves, even while sitting quietly on a cushion. When we first begin a meditation practice, the technique itself can feel interesting and entertaining but that soon fades. Following this honeymoon period, you are more likely to experience the cool boredom that naturally arises as the result of *not* filling in spaces and *not* reacting to your reaction, positive or negative. Whether on your meditation cushion or in your life, think of boredom as an invitation to be with yourself. To befriend whatever is happening in your mind, body, and heart in that moment. A willingness to be bored is an integral part of both meditation and the Eat to Love path.

When do you find yourself eating out of boredom? How can you work with this obstacle? How might you reframe this experience with compassion?

Emotional Overeating

No matter how clear our intention to eat according to internal physical sensations and how consistently we practice, there may be times we eat more out of emotional than physical hunger. This too is not a problem. We all encounter difficulty and struggle at times. How we respond to those times depends on a lot of variables, including physical health, wellness, or illness; whether we are getting enough sleep and water; whether we are feeding ourselves adequately and regularly; whether we are getting enough intimacy and emotional support; and how much stress we are under.

It is helpful to remind ourselves that beneath our emotional overeating is a desire to feel okay. Even if it has become a habitual and dysfunctional behavior, overeating emotionally might have worked in some way in the past when it was simply the best that we could do. For these reasons, we must meet our emotional overeating with gentleness and compassion rather than self-criticism, aggression, and feelings of defeat. Only when we learn to turn toward our difficulty with gentleness rather than aggression do we discover its origins and begin to move toward better means of working with them.

Our willingness to meet ourselves where we are is also likely to transform our relationship with this habitual behavior. The more we create space for whatever thoughts and feelings arise, the less relief emotional overeating actually provides. Initially this feels like a loss, but it is evidence of your courage and progress.

When do you find yourself overeating emotionally? How can you work with this obstacle? How might you reframe this experience with compassion?

Substituting Food for Intimacy

One particular form of emotional overeating is substituting food for intimacy. Intimacy could be a deep, meaningful friendship, a romantic involvement, or a purely sensual relationship. Even though we all need intimacy to live rich, satisfying lives, the fact that it involves other human beings sometimes makes it feel, shall we say, complicated. The vulnerability inherent in intimate relationships makes them simultaneously powerful and terrifying. The stakes are higher when you care and when you genuinely reveal yourself to others. Food, by contrast, feels uncomplicated: an easier route to pleasure, sensuality, and indulgence. When we eat in private, safe from outside judgment, there is no fear of awkwardness, rejection, or heartbreak. Yet food will never truly substitute for intimacy.

To work with this obstacle, practice noticing it with great compassion. Once you have identified it, acknowledge whatever fears, anxieties, or past experiences prevent you from reaching out to other people as your heart desires. If possible, turn toward and really feel the sadness, longing, sorrow, or any other emotion that exists beneath the fear. Do this for as little or as long as you wish.

When do you find yourself substituting food for intimacy? How can you work with this obstacle? How might you reframe this experience with compassion?

Switching from Inhabiting Your Body to Looking at Your Body from the Outside

Even as we become more comfortable fully inhabiting our bodies and making self-care decisions from that internal perspective, sometimes something jolts us and causes us to change perspective, whether it's during some form of physical activity, a triggering aspect of diet culture, compare and despair behavior, or suddenly thinking negative or critical thoughts about our bodies. When something specific, or seemingly nothing in particular, causes you to shift from inhabiting your body and making decisions from the inside to looking at yourself critically from the outside, acknowledge what has happened as soon as you notice. Identify what provoked you to take this outside-looking-in perspective with nonjudgmental curiosity. And gently shift back to being inside your body by emphasizing your senses of sight, smell, hearing, and touch. This practice helps us to acknowledge lingering self-aggressive thoughts and behaviors, renounce them, and keep coming back to our bodies in the moment. Rather than spending time feeling bad about ourselves, trying to fix ourselves, or treating ourselves as problems, we see ourselves honestly: wonderfully imperfect, constantly changing beings working with whatever arises moment to moment.

When do you notice you have shifted to being outside your body? How can you work with this obstacle? How might you reframe this experience with compassion?

Feeling Nostalgia for Magical Eating

Even though the Eat to Love approach is based on kindness, compassion, and our actual needs, at times we might miss elements of magical eating and long for the excitement and hopefulness of starting a new diet even though it was short-lived. We may miss its sense of control, however illusory, and wish to feel the certainty about the future when our new, thinner bodies would finally make us happy, even though part of us probably knew that was too good to be true.

Sadness often underlies nostalgia. A grieving process may naturally follow renouncing magical eating. When you have cycled through diet after diet and come to the realization that they are based in insanity, their rewarding qualities diminish. Even if we are tempted to regress to magical eating, our new awareness eventually undercuts what previously motivated us to deprive ourselves and treat our bodies with aggression.

Feeling nostalgia for old habits is a normal part of any big change. Acknowledging our feelings still permits us to continue on the path, coming back to the body, discovering what we are feeling, discerning what we need the most, and taking the next step. Our nostalgia need not derail our progress. And such thoughts need not be squashed (this is just another form of self-aggression). When all thoughts and feelings are welcome, we continue to work with what is and move toward wellness defined by mindfulness and awareness.

When do you feel nostalgia for magical eating? How can you work with this obstacle? How might you reframe this experience with compassion?

Obstacles arise to teach us something essential. If whatever happens on our unique Eat to Love path is exactly what needs to happen, the only real mishap is wanting things to be different. The antidote to any resistance, and the antidote to all obstacles, is practicing the paramita of patience.

The next slogan supports our practice of patience by reminding us that whatever we encounter enriches our path. Our challenges are essential to deepening our self-understanding. Without them, we don't learn anything. Moments of progress also deepen our self-knowing. Without them, we don't see the trend toward positive change and peace with food and our bodies.

Whatever you meet unexpectedly, join with meditation

As you recognize the various aspects of your experience, whatever strikes you, surprises you, pleases you, and disrupts you, join them with meditation by allowing these insights to arise, level off, and dissolve without attachment. Just watch them as you do any thought that arises in shamatha meditation. As with the practice of tranquility, let your mind's awareness ride the waves of the breath and come back any time that strays, without reacting automatically, until it is clear what action is necessary (or whether any action is necessary). There is no need to be seated on a cushion or chair when you do this. It is meditation in action, a way of working with your actual life.

What is a challenge you worked through on your Eat to Love path? What did you learn from it? What is a challenge you are currently working through? What are you learning from it?

Our meditation practice supports our ability to recognize and work with obstacles with patience and self-compassion. The tools we need to practice meditation—our bodies, hearts, and minds—are always with us.

THE PARAMITA

OF EXERTION

XERTION IS HOW we maintain a connection with the Eat to Love path through its inevitable ups and downs. It comprises trust and continual effort united with self-care, compassion, and the desire to be of benefit to others. When you maintain a strong connection with your Eat to Love path, rather than being deceived by the shiny newness of a diet, you derive joy and motivation from clearly seeing yourself, your thoughts, and your behaviors. Unlike diets, which are static and do not adapt to changing needs, the Eat to Love approach evolves with you so that each day, each meal, and each bite is appreciated as unique.

A key difference between the Eat to Love path and a diet, whether or not it is expressly called that, is that our approach lasts a lifetime, while a diet occupies a temporary period marked by a brief and predictable lifespan. Diets begin with a desire to be thin, to eat clean, or to rid the body of fat and toxins, but underneath all of that, we now understand, is some form of dis-ease that we attempt to cure by manipulating our bodies. This desire for mastery fuels an eating style driven by external systems while neglecting the intelligence of the body. The misguided deference to experts and diets induces the negative effects of physical and emotional deprivation. Ferocious hunger and irresistible cravings inevitably lead to overeating, causing weight regain, weight cycling, remorse, and feelings of failure.

Ultimately this leads you back to where you began, wishing to be thin, to eat clean, or to rid the body of fat and toxins.

As insane and redundant as this cycle is, there are elements that are appealing. Those first few days of a new diet feel exciting and full of potential, sort of like falling in love. Even if you feel deprived, your hopeful anticipation propels you forward. Seeing initial results like losing a few pounds rationalizes the cost. But as the novelty subsides and is replaced with frustration, impatience, and despondency, you lose your motivation and even swing toward the opposite extreme by overeating, binging, and not taking caring of yourself, even in enjoyable ways, because there is no promise of weight loss. An approach that is sustainable over the course of your life, on the other hand, requires a new view to feel inspiring and hopeful over the long term.

Exertion is the absence of laziness. It requires an ongoing infusion of energy motivated by our true desires and deepest values. We all experience laziness sometimes, and this is not a problem. Consider it one more obstacle with the potential to deepen our commitment to and understanding of ourselves. In Buddhist thought, there are three kinds of laziness: ordinary laziness, disheartenment, and becoming too busy. Each of the three types has an antidote, which makes laziness very workable.

The first, ordinary laziness, is exactly what you think: not bringing a sense of joy and energy to what you do because of a lack of mindfulness and precise attention. The antidote to ordinary laziness is to reinvigorate your mindfulness practice by sharpening your attention, reconnecting with the senses, and coming back to the body again and again. This might mean reminding yourself why you are pursuing this path, what experiences brought you here, and why it is worth the effort to work with your body through your Eat to Love path and with your mind through your meditation practice. It could be a time to review the costs of magical eating on page 108. Your lived experience is the greatest teacher. And your body as it is right now serves as your main point of reference. Coming back to it and asking what it needs is how you maintain the strong connection of exertion. In applying the antidote to ordinary laziness, the superficial novelty of diets is replaced by the true novelty of always being able to take a fresh start.

When do you experience ordinary laziness on your Eat to Love path? How can you apply the antidote?

The second kind of laziness, disheartenment, arises when you lose faith in the process and resign yourself to the status quo, thinking, *What's the point?* In choosing the Eat to Love path and beginning to work with uncomfortable emotions rather than anesthetizing them with food, you might even feel things are getting worse! Emotions that drove you to overeat could seem to increase in severity. Plus, many people feel lonely traveling such a counterculture path while everyone else continues to bang their heads against the magical eating wall without question. Never knowing for sure if you're doing it right may lead to disheartenment and a nostalgia for magical eating, which, even if it was oppressive, at least clearly defined right and wrong. Perfectionism and the failure to sustain a flawless Eat to Love path (which is totally not the point) is a special kind of disheartenment that disorients us and makes us want to give up. Recognizing how difficult it is to feel the full range of our emotions and change the way we relate to them may feel supremely disheartening. The antidote to disheartenment is to acknowledge it, allow yourself to feel it, rebalance your perspective by appreciating your accomplishments, and reconnect with your values.

Working with disheartenment does not mean never having negative feelings about this process. Instead of squashing them, acknowledge and feel them and still treat yourself with kindness. Whenever you notice doubt, anger, sadness, loneliness, or longing, acknowledge it out loud or in writing and feel it until it shifts or morphs or leaves on its own; it always does. Treat it as you would any thought that arises during your meditation practice, or, as Shunryu Suzuki Roshi said, "Leave your front door and your back door open. Allow your thoughts to come and go. Just don't serve them tea." Knowing it will not last allows us to ride it out.

As you feel uncomfortable emotions, also remember the progress you've made, from the moment you first questioned magical eating to identifying how you internalized it in even the subtlest ways, and gradually moving toward feeding yourself compassionately. Celebrating even the smallest points of progress reminds you how far you have come, serves as a counterbalance to disheartenment, and helps you see the gradual but significant positive trend. When you do notice evidence of progress, recall how that growth was underway when you weren't fully aware of it, perhaps even during a time you felt disheartened. When difficulty or stagnation arises, imagine that something is coming into fruition that just isn't ready to harvest yet. Then, when disheartenment comes to visit, it doesn't stay long.

Once you have felt your disheartenment and reminded yourself of the progress you have made, reconnect with the things you care about. Most of us value playing with our kids, walking the dogs, being in nature, walking on the beach, or cooking a delectable meal and not feeling ill afterward. Connecting (and reconnecting as often as you need to) with your deepest values leads you to take a bigger view. Acknowledging our frustrations and challenges, celebrating our progress and victories, and reconnecting with our deepest values allows us to see more clearly what is happening, where we are coming from, and the direction in which we are moving.

When do you experience disheartenment? What does it look and feel like for you? What are points of progress that you can call up when feeling disheartened? What are your values that are consistent with staying on the Eat to Love path?

The third kind of laziness, becoming too busy, is when everything else takes precedence over our efforts to care for ourselves, whether that is work, housework, reality television, social media, or the needs of family, friends, and countless others. The antidote to being too busy is to review your priorities. When it has become the norm to care for everyone and everything before meeting your own needs, you default to a survival mode in which eating, drinking water, sleeping, and other aspects of self-care take a back seat.

We are only genuinely of benefit to others when our own basic needs are met. We only authentically treat others with kindness and compassion when we first offer those things to ourselves. To quote the safety instructions on any airplane that has ever left the ground, "Please put on your own oxygen mask before helping others." Experiencing the laziness of being too busy is a good time to come back to the paramita of generosity and why our basically good bodies deserve our care.

When do you experience the laziness of being too busy? How can you apply the antidote?

Throughout the course of your Eat to Love path, it is likely that you will experience all three kinds of laziness at some point. This is not a problem.

ERICA GREW UP with a dieting mom and was always doing magical eating of a sort. She and her mom often dieted together and learned how to support one another to stick with ridiculous regimens. Later, at the age of thirty-three, Erica worked in a busy law firm among colleagues who habitually disregarded their basic needs for food, water, and sleep, yet managed to get up at 5 a.m. for grueling workouts. Erica and I worked together to dispel her magical eating beliefs and help her shift her allegiance back to the intelligence of her body. During that time, she went through a number of ups and downs, seasons, holidays, and phases of self-care, including the three kinds of laziness. One of the biggest barriers to taking consistent care of herself was Erica's job, which was either extremely demanding or on hyperdrive. She often worked nights and weekends and her capacity to recognize and respond to her body's needs suffered. When work occasionally slowed down, it felt easier to lounge on the couch instead of seizing the opportunity to take better care of herself. In response to this first kind of laziness, sometimes Erica gave herself permission to just be lazy, while other times she decided to revisit the goals we had established at the beginning of our work together—to not get too hungry, to respect her tastes and desires, and to reprioritize embodied movement—and took what steps she could to meet those goals. When work became absolutely overwhelming and these goals again took a backseat to the needs of her firm, she created a weekly ritual of food shopping and prep that ensured her a week's worth of satisfying lunches that met her taste and energy needs (even though it was never perfect). When even this was impossible, she gave herself permission to experiment with take-out from different places.

Because of Erica's history of deprivation, it took some time to feel she could trust her body and also feel satisfied. At times, she bypassed comfortable fullness because part of her still believed she would not have consistent access to her favorite foods. As a result, she gained some weight. When Erica became disheartened, our work shifted to feeling her sadness and disappointment, understanding more fully how she felt losing weight would make her life better, and revisiting past session notes to mark her progress. At one of our appointments near Hanukkah, we looked back at the previous holiday season and found that Erica had been much more fearful about all the foods that would be available and anxious about her mom's comments about her eating or her weight. This Hanukkah, however, she was looking forward to her favorite foods, had a conversation with her mom about how to support her, and felt confident in her body and its intelligence (as well as in the new clothes she had purchased that were comfortable and showed her own style).

Even once we have addressed the different forms of laziness, bringing energy and motivation to our Eat to Love path over the long term is challenging. Because the Eat to Love path is a long and somewhat unpredictable one, having a framework to reinvigorate our practice helps us continually re-engage and remember why we practice.

Practice the five strengths, the condensed heart instruction

The five strengths described in this slogan are: strong determination, familiarization, seed of virtue, reproach, and aspiration. Let's take a closer look at each of the five strengths and how they help bring exertion to your ongoing Eat to Love path.

Strong Determination

Having strong determination means connecting with your intentions in looking at your mind, continually evaluating your relationship with food and body, and committing to steps that align with deeper values of compassion, kindness, and being of benefit to others. One way to practice strong determination is to begin every morning by reaffirming your commitment to this path; to remind yourself why you are caring for your body as it is today, so that you feel well, worthy, and whole and can ultimately fulfill your potential in being of benefit to others. You could say something silently to yourself such as, *May I meet what today offers by caring for myself to the best of my ability, by making nourishing choices for my body and mind, so that I am part of positive change in my own life and in the lives of others.*

Bring to mind your strong determination every night by reviewing the day and noticing if you were able to maintain your intention or if doing so became difficult or impossible. If you were able to maintain your intention, inquire what made this possible. If you were not able to maintain your intention, forgive yourself and become curious about what made it more difficult. By bookending your day with setting an intention and reviewing it, you become intertwined with your strong determination. It becomes like a beloved who always fills your heart with joy.

How can you reaffirm your commitment to your own Eat to Love path each morning? In reviewing your commitment at the end of the day, what makes it easier to maintain? What makes it more difficult?

Familiarization

In the second of the five strengths, we practice familiarization. This means remembering how all aspects of your life, all the ways in which you nourish yourself and care for your body, should be brought to the path. There is no separation between you and your Eat to Love path. It is familiar and intimate and, therefore, completely integrated into your life. Even as you meet obstacles and challenges, you keep coming back. As you learned in the previous chapter on patience, obstacles are not considered problems but instead essential teachers. In the chapter on discipline, you examined the possibility of seeing new thought patterns and behaviors as "side paths" that are reinforced by recognizing the transformation point and choosing it again and again, gradually shifting you toward desired ways of thinking and behaving.

There has always been something delightful about the willingness to become familiar with all aspects of our experience. Particularly when it concerns food and body, we have a tendency to be very problem-solution oriented. By practicing familiarization, before we even come to see something as a problem, we give ourselves the opportunity to feel it.

MONICA IS A veterinarian who always felt different from her family and friends. From the time she was a child, she was more sensitive than her peers and indeed her parents, who had a tendency to pathologize her sensitivity and sent her to all manner of child psychologists. Because her dad (who was the sole breadwinner) held an unpredictable job, her family went through phases of feast or famine. Monica occasionally went hungry. She learned to fear the physical sensation of hunger because of its association with neglect and danger. When Monica responded physically and emotionally to her extreme hunger, her parents downplayed the effect that it had on her, which caused her to feel she could trust neither her body nor her mind. As Monica grew into an older child, teenager, and then young woman, she tried every diet she heard of to master her appetite and control her body. The inevitable physical and psychological deprivation that resulted led Monica to binge, which only solidified her belief that she needed more self-control. The first time I spoke to Monica, she shared the cycle she found herself in. She went from feeling bad about her body to looking at "thinspiration" pictures, pinching her body where she felt any flesh, and restricting her food to feel in control. This inevitably led to losing control and binging. The binging part of her cycle lasted anywhere from a few days to several weeks, after which she would come back to feeling bad about her body and start the whole thing all over again.

As we worked together, we began to understand Monica's cycle in more depth. Through refraining from treating the individual stages of the cycle as problems to be diagnosed and fixed, Monica learned to stay with her experience and get familiar with the nuances of what each part of her cycle felt like. We discovered that any threat to her security, real or imagined, caused her to double down on efforts to control her body, that her desire to please others above all led her to punish herself with how she used food, and that internalization of the weight stigma she learned in her home community taught her to value smaller bodies over bigger ones. When I first introduced the concept of developing friendliness toward the pieces of her experience that felt most painful, Monica laughed out loud. "Sorry, but that's crazy" is what she said to me, I believe. But she later commented that it was familiarizing herself with what she previously thought intolerable that helped her see the cause-and-effect nature of her cycle and interrupt its momentum.

What do your cycles of magical eating look like? Practice familiarization with your own eating and body image thoughts.

Seed of Virtue

The third of the five strengths is the seed of virtue. This means using our minds, speech, and bodies to plant seeds that eventually ripen as compassion, gentleness, and understanding. The significance of the word "seed" is that even the tiniest actions, words, and thoughts have value and importance in moving us toward peace. Nothing is too small to matter if it is done with the intentions we set with strong determination and the sense of integration we establish with familiarization.

Sometimes it will feel effortless to plant seeds of virtue. Other times it will feel more difficult. It is easier to maintain a positive state of mind when internal and external stress levels are lower, when we are gentle with ourselves, and when our experiences don't strengthen the grip of magical eating. When we find it more challenging to maintain a positive outlook, on the other hand, because we are sick or emotionally stressed, we plant a seed of virtue by reconnecting with the intention to treat ourselves gently, with kindness and compassion. Doing so makes it much easier to find our way back to a positive outlook than if we were to treat ourselves harshly.

It is only through acknowledging the smallest actions, words, and thoughts that we ultimately appreciate the overall trend toward creating a gentler relationship with food and our bodies. Here are some questions to ask yourself to plant the seeds of virtue to establish and maintain a loving and compassionate relationship with food and your body.

How can I compassionately work with my thoughts today? How can I speak to myself and others with gentleness today? What small actions can I take to show myself care today? What small actions can I take with others to plant seeds of virtue today?

How can I use my body as an instrument rather than treat it as an object today? What helps me see the value of even the smallest aspect of my Eat to Love path?

Reproach

The fourth strength is reproach, which means acknowledging the subtle yet widespread damage done by magical eating. Practicing reproach comprises exposing the "alternative facts" of the diet culture, how it has hurt both you personally and the wider circle of other women (and men and children). It also means accepting and seeing clearly how you internalized magical eating and used it to be harsh, critical, and aggressive toward yourself and perhaps also toward others. By practicing reproach, we willingly see the deceptions of the diet culture and how they have distorted what it means to take care of ourselves and to treat ourselves with respect, thereby causing us to deceive and harm ourselves.

Reproach toward the diet culture and magical eating may take many forms both big and small. Allowing ourselves to sit comfortably in a chair rather than positioning ourselves to take up as little space as possible, and dressing well and comfortably rather than in a way that is considered flattering or slimming. Presenting ourselves in a way that is pleasing to ourselves rather than camouflaging or concealing what others consider negative or unattractive, and participating in activities that feel good in our bodies without concern for how we look to others.

Reproach may also manifest as a form of anti–magical eating activism. Like *not* contributing to the $66-billion diet industry; not patronizing the guerilla marketers for fashion, beauty products, and anything targeting our vulnerabilities; changing how we engage with the social media machines of Facebook, Twitter, Instagram, and beyond; and changing how we consume magical eating propaganda such as retouched photos and incompletely represented before-and-after stories. Directly calling out bias in all its forms and condemning discrimination based on sex, age, race, culture, sexual orientation, gender identity, wealth, status, ability, and body size. Every day it is possible to practice reproach by asking ourselves, *What can I do today to make the world kinder and more compassionate and to disrupt magical eating and biases of all kinds?*

What do you notice now (that perhaps you didn't before) about the effects of magical eating? How can you disrupt magical eating in your own life and in the larger culture?

Aspiration

The fifth strength is aspiration, or connecting with the desire to alleviate the suffering caused by magical eating to both yourself and others. Practicing aspiration takes many forms but one simple way is to dedicate the merit of everything we do on this path to the benefit of all beings (which, by the way, includes ourselves). Dedicating the merit at the end of our meditation practice is a wonderful way to practice this. Dedicating the merit of any aspect of our Eat to Love path also has tremendous value—when we catch ourselves going down a habitual pathway, whether we choose to continue down that path or to try something new; when we notice even a tiny point of progress; when we do something with the mind of generosity, discipline, patience, exertion, meditation, or wisdom; when we do something to disrupt the diet culture in a skillful way; or when we simply treat ourselves or others with kindness and compassion. Even when we taste the perfect bite of food.

All thoughts, words, and actions have merit that may be dedicated in the service of our aspiration. You could say something like, *May my intentions, words, and actions on my own Eat to Love path to making peace with food and my body help others so that they may also find this clarity, gentleness, and compassion.* We may not know how our intentions, words, and deeds are actually of benefit to others but we continue to practice this by wishing that others too wake up rather than further solidify habitual and destructive thoughts and behaviors.

How can you dedicate the merit of your Eat to Love practice and your words, thoughts, and actions?

Bringing exertion to your Eat to Love path is a daily practice of returning to your heart and body, revisiting the values that brought you here, and continually reinvigorating your thoughts, speech, and actions with energy and connection. By working with the three forms of laziness and practicing the five strengths of strong determination, familiarization, seed of virtue, reproach, and aspiration, our Eat to Love path remains a dynamic and engaged process of working with what is, so that it grows and changes with us.

THE PARAMITA

OF MEDITATION

THE MINDFULNESS MOVEMENT is a wonderful thing. Whenever we bring our full attention to what we are doing, the result is genuine and beneficial. But as mindfulness has become more mainstream, meditation is often left out, suggesting that just paying closer attention to our daily activities is a shortcut to inner peace. After years of investigation, I disagree. Mindfulness without meditation is like a fat-free cupcake: hard, dense, and lacking in tenderness. Similarly, attempting to travel your Eat to Love path without a meditation practice is likely to be short-lived and without depth. You may read the book, do the contemplations, and change your intellectual understanding of magical eating. That is all wonderful! But until you begin to work with your mind through the practice of meditation (even if you begin with tiny, imperfect steps; full instructions available on page 55, by the way), you will only go so far. As you learned in chapter 2, meditation changes both the structure and function of the brain in ways that affect our lives on and off the cushion. And as my meditation teacher says, "We don't practice meditation to become good at meditating; we practice meditation to become good at life."

I know this from experience. After a painful breakup and while I was still wondering whether I had a drinking problem, a friend recommended *The Places That Scare You* by Pema Chödrön. This was before I had begun a personal meditation practice and long before I became a Buddhist, but the title spoke to me so I bought and read it. It was immediately clear that the wisdom in that book had everything to do with what I was going through (and what we all go through). She touched on something I had had an inkling of since childhood but could never put into words: becoming more comfortable with discomfort might just be the most important thing we ever do. I was particularly struck by the idea that it is not by changing our negative emotions that we liberate ourselves, but rather it is by staying with them and relating to them directly that we change how we experience them. Throughout the book, she refers to meditation as the foundation for cultivating this wisdom. But even though I hung on her every word, I wasn't ready to sit down and meditate yet. Instead I tried to apply Chödrön's explanation of life to my own, which as it turned out was only so useful.

Years later, after I had begun my own meditation practice, I came back to this book and found it to be completely different. Having begun to work with my own mind through meditation changed the way I understood everything, particularly how to relate to the most difficult and uncomfortable aspects of my life, such as why I had used alcohol and why I had continued to use other behaviors like dieting, emotional overeating, shopping, and even habitual thoughts to avoid suffering. Whether during times of difficulty or smooth sailing, the people in my life started to notice that I was becoming calmer and more resilient. No less emotional, but more able to ride the ups and downs.

Though the first time I read her book, I revered Pema Chödrön as the authority on what was right for me, coming back to it after beginning a meditation practice my perception was very different; learning to sit with myself helped me see that no one else on the planet was a better judge of what was going on for me, with me, and in me than me.

By training us to become more comfortable with discomfort, meditation is like exposure therapy for our lives. Rather than transcending the human condition and dodging suffering, meditation allows us to experience our lives without a filter and to become more authentically ourselves. It is a practice of allowing ourselves to be as we are without trying to change and with a willingness to work with whatever arises.

Our meditation practice is actually the foundation upon which we apply the other paramitas. A meditation practice makes it possible to connect with the unborn awareness of the senses, to shift our allegiance from external systems to internal sensations of how to eat, and to offer ourselves and others the gifts of ordinary generosity, fearlessness, and sharing the dharma. Meditation slows things down so that we discover the true nature of our bodies, hearts, and minds, and we are able to practice the discipline of discerning what is actually happening from moment to moment so that we may respond skillfully and precisely. Sitting in meditation softens our hearts and allows us to relate directly to strong emotions with openness, curiosity, and a sense of friendliness, and to speak to ourselves with compassion as we work with the obstacles that naturally arise on the path. And it alerts us whenever we need to reconnect with our Eat to Love path with energy, motivation, and exertion. As you will see in the next chapter on wisdom, meditation also supports our understanding of how to thoughtfully re-integrate some of the information from outside ourselves into our self-care. Put simply: meditation is the core practice for the warrior bodhisattva.

Pema Chödrön has said, "Meditation practice isn't about trying to throw ourselves away and become something better; it's about befriending who we are already." Those who promote magical eating have profited enormously from the assertion that we should throw ourselves away and become something else. That we cannot trust our own bodies and minds to know and do what is right. Magical eating teaches us that if left to our own devices, we would eat chocolate cake and cheeseburgers day in and day out, never do any kind of physical movement, and be unhealthy and unloved. The fear of these consequences led us to willingly, if fearfully, hand over our allegiance and trust to something or someone outside our own bodies and minds. Having an Eat to Love practice in which we cultivate a compassionate and peaceful relationship with food and our bodies means taking that power back and relying on ourselves first and foremost as the decision makers. We befriend ourselves by becoming loyal to our own perspective.

Of the two witnesses, hold the principal one

In any situation, there is your own perspective (the principal perspective) and the perspective of anyone who isn't you, whether that is magical eating thoughts, a supposed health expert, or a well-meaning doctor, dietitian, family member, or friend. By asking us to hold the principal witness, this slogan asks us to trust our own insight over that of anyone else. We are the only one who knows what is going on in our bodies and minds. We are the only expert in what we need. We are the only one who accurately experiences ourselves as we are: not to find problems to fix, but to witness ourselves without delusion. Based on this pure perception, only we know whether we are moving toward being gentle, open, and compassionate with ourselves and toward treating our bodies with generosity, discipline, patience, exertion, and wisdom.

Our meditation practice is the most important tool in learning to hold the principal witness. In shamatha meditation, the practice of tranquility, we substitute for our discursive mind another object of attention. That object is the breath, something that is always accessible and always in the present moment. As we feel the breath, we take a comfortable, upright posture that balances relaxation with upliftedness. We allow the mind to settle but do not try to clear it or change the thoughts we are thinking. We simply let them be as they are, placing thought in the *background* of our attention while feeling the breath in the *foreground*. Finally, we train our minds to recognize whenever we have become absorbed in thought and then to gently and precisely bring our attention back to the breath.

Instead of requiring us to stop thinking or to only think pleasant thoughts, which would be a form of self-aggression and a recipe for frustration, we are permitted to be as we are. In allowing our minds to be as they are without trying to change them, we create space that allows us to relate with thoughts differently. In this space, we begin to notice what arises without judgment or habitual reactions. In the spirit of the teaching that you can never receive too much meditation instruction, please review the extensive meditation instruction on page 55 as well as what follows.

Come to a comfortable seated position, whether on the floor with your legs crossed loosely in front of you or in a chair with your feet flat on the floor. Allow the lower body to feel heavy and rooted into the ground while the upper body feels light and reaches gently upward. The strength of the back supports your posture while the softness of the front body allows you to be open and receptive. Relax the shoulders down the back and let the hands rest palms down on the tops of the legs. Release all the little muscles in the face, neck, and throat. Let the eyes be open and soft with a gaze that is cast down at a distance of about six feet in front of you, and breathe normally in and out through the nose.

Feel the breath. Have a sense of accompanying the breath as it comes in through the nostrils and fills your lungs and then dissolves out of your body and into the space around you. You might even imagine being the breath itself. Let your mind's awareness ride the full cycle of the breath through each inhale and exhale, staying with it to the best of your ability, noticing that thoughts continue to pop up, flicker, or pass by and that most come and go on their own if we don't get attached to them.

Notice the quality of the mind that you have brought to your meditation practice in this moment. Is it stormy? Speedy? Placid? Dreamy? Worried? Silly? Note the texture of your thoughts. Are they sharp? Soft? Dull? Spiky? Tight? Loose? Changeable?

Notice what you encounter when you place your mind's awareness on the feeling of the breath. How does it feel to maintain this connection? What does it feel like when you lose it? What was the sequence of events leading you to become absorbed in thought?

Practice this technique of placing the feeling of the breath in the foreground while everything else rests in the background for a few minutes before bringing your practice to a close.

For many of us, when we sit down and attempt to place our body and mind in the same place at the same time to meditate, we realize how difficult this is. Our bodies are not the culprits here. They are always in the present moment. Our hearts beat, blood pumps, lungs breathe, eyes and ears see and hear, always now. Our minds, on the other hand, are less reliably present. While meditating, we place our attention on the feeling of the breath, which is always happening in the present moment, yet our minds have a tendency to wander, to seek entertainment, and to be anywhere but here. They might be somewhere in the past, replaying memories, revisiting old joys or regrets, or wishing something turned out differently than it did. Or off in the future, making to-do lists, thinking about lunch, planning your next vacation, or just daydreaming. Even watching the candle flicker on the table in front of you or imagining cartoon characters out of the whorls of the wood floorboards could seem preferable to staying with your actual experience in the moment. (Or maybe that's just me.)

Whenever we realize we have abandoned the breath and become absorbed in thought, whether we have been there mere seconds or the majority of our sit, we apply the technique of letting the thought go with precision and gently bringing our attention back to the breath. No matter the content of the thought—good, bad, boring, sad, brilliant, dull, and every possibility in between—or how many times we notice we have lost that attention on the object of our meditation, we come back and take a fresh start. Noticing that we have gotten lost is a moment of wakefulness, a moment of clear-seeing. To the outside observer, meditation looks as if we are doing nothing. But this is a very active process. Applying the meditation technique means we are constantly staying with the various shifts, energies, and moods our minds go through and not reacting.

One way to work toward non-reactivity is when you notice an itch during your meditation practice. Our natural instinct is to immediately relieve discomfort by scratching. But to become more mindful of reactions to different stimuli, rather than immediately scratching, just sit with the itch and pay attention to it. Where is it exactly? How does it feel? Does it change from one moment to the next? Does it go away and come back? Does it shift to some other body part? Similarly, treat your thoughts this way by pausing to notice how they feel (not what they mean) before letting them go and coming back to the breath.

Just as we pause before reacting habitually to an itch or a thought while meditating, we pause before we react physically or emotionally to magical eating triggers. Taking a few moments to pay attention to exactly how a small discomfort feels helps us learn more about the way we think and respond to different situations. Turning fully toward our discomfort takes an enormous amount of courage but actually is a lot less scary than pushing it away with food or other substances. As we develop the capacity to tolerate our own emotional discomfort, it increases our connection with others who inevitably also suffer and struggle. In this way, we lessen our own isolation, as well as that of others, and deepen our compassion for self and others.

What has stopped you from trusting your body and judgment? How does it feel to hold the principal witness in your meditation practice? How do you normally respond to discomfort? What might it feel like to stay with that discomfort?

The Eat to Love path is dynamic and constantly changing. Meditation is the best support to recognizing change as it is occurring and being able to pivot as needed to continue to meet our needs. What I have observed in the clients I work with who have a meditation practice is that they are generally more finely attuned to these changes than those who do not. The meditators see themselves more clearly, without delusion, without diminishing any part of their experience and without exaggerating it. They sense shifts as they are happening, sometimes even anticipating them based on the insight gained from past experiences, and are able to continually assess the changing needs of their bodies, hearts, and minds. Ultimately they discern what qualities to bring to their practice, whether that is generosity, discipline, patience, exertion, or wisdom.

ASHLEY BEGAN A meditation practice a few months into our work together. At that time, she was struggling with nightly emotional overeating and body image concerns, including avoiding her reflection in the mirror and covering her body in long sleeves and long pants, even on vacation in warm climates. She never allowed certain foods into her home for fear she would eat them all, was fixated on losing weight, and did not believe her body would find a natural weight if she ate as she wanted.

Over the course of more than a year, Ashley and I worked to honor the information coming from her intelligent body, including noticing when she was physically hungry, eating what she was truly hungry for, and experimenting with stopping as she noticed her body becoming satisfied. When she craved certain foods in the absence of physical hunger, we reinforced absolute permission and ensured she had an ample supply of her favorite ice cream in the freezer at all times. During this time, Ashley continued her some-times-inconsistent meditation practice, began reading a dharma book about relationships, and attended several talks at a local meditation center.

Directly and indirectly, Ashley began to see the connection between her progress and her meditation practice. Slowing things down and recognizing when she was at a transformation point, feeling more able to stay with difficult emotions, and simply feeling what was happening in her body in real time solidified both her meditation and her Eat to Love practice.

As Ashley continued to meditate and trust her body's intelligence, she amassed a collection of experiences in which she ate what she wanted, when she was hungry, to the point of satisfaction but not discomfort. Though she continued to struggle with body image, even as her weight gradually went down, she also began to experiment with her own personal style, including more dresses, sleeveless tops, and one-piece bathing suits. She became more tolerant and accepting of strong emotions and rarely emotionally overate. As of our last session, Ashley had had the same three pints of her favorite ice cream in her freezer for several weeks.

As we continue on the Eat to Love path, our thinking about food, eating, and body evolves. What began as obsession slowly becomes focused and thoughtful awareness. Though it might feel like you are experiencing the same quantity of thoughts about food and body with awareness as you did with obsession, the quality of your thoughts shifts from distressful to spacious. Finally, awareness transforms into integrated mindfulness in which parts of this process feel like second nature. Our meditation practice on the cushion and our practice in relating to food, our bodies, and our surroundings off the cushion are happening all the time, even when we are not paying full attention. And because the Eat to Love path is still somewhat counterculture, there are many distractions that could cause you to question yourself.

If you can practice even when distracted, you are well trained

In describing this lojong slogan, many people use the analogy of a horseback rider. As she becomes more and more seasoned, she may allow her mind to wander without falling off her horse. When how you work with your mind aligns with how you feed your body, your Eat to Love practice begins to be more fully integrated into your everyday life. So you may not need to concentrate as much on shifting your allegiance. It will happen again and again in a more natural way. Going out to dinner with friends, eating popcorn while watching a movie, or grabbing a snack on the go contain within them the recognition of and response to internal sensations of hunger, fullness, preference, and satisfaction.

At the same time, changing our relationship with food and body is not a quick or linear process. Every seeming slip is not a failure but a signal to come back to our bodies in the present moment with self-compassion. If, during a meal with your partner, the conversation gets heated and you find yourself eating in an emotional way, that moment serves as a call to pay attention, be gentle, and respond skillfully to what you determine to be your need at that time.

Perhaps the biggest distraction to our Eat to Love practice is uncertainty. Though past diets never perfectly aligned with our actual and constantly changing needs, they seemed so solid and certain in how they prescribed specific round numbers of calories or grams of fat and simplified weight loss to an easy math equation. Diets gave us definite guidelines to measure our progress and quantify success or failure. The Eat to Love approach lacks such certainty because, in reality, it does not exist. In working with your present needs of hunger, fullness, and satisfaction, you use your best judgment but may never be 100 percent certain that your decisions are the right ones. Accepting this uncertainty is essential to learning to trust yourself long term. How you know is through having the willingness to make decisions based on your good-enough awareness and self-understanding in the moment and then compassionately evaluating how those decisions worked for you. Though you won't get the same black-and-white reassurance you got from magical eating, what you will get is much more valuable: self-trust, flexibility, and resilience.

Even though we are creating a new way of relating to our bodies that is kind, gentle, and geared toward using them as instruments of our lives, there will be moments that the harmful narrative weasels its way back into your mind. This is also not a problem. Having occasional negative thoughts and feelings about your body is completely normal. Many people respond to negative thoughts by trying to cut them off, silence them, or stop thinking altogether. This is just another form of self-aggression. In our practice, we make room for all thoughts. When you notice you are having negative thoughts, you turn toward them with a sense of friendliness. Just as you do in your meditation practice, touch the thought lightly with your mind and then let it go.

Or perhaps respond to the negative thought with a more neutral or even self-compassionate one, as described in the chapter on patience.

The most basic way to work with distractions is always to come back to the body. Just as the breath serves as the object of your meditation practice, the body serves as the object of your Eat to Love practice. Whenever you realize you have become absorbed in grasping, aggression, ignorance, fantasy, worrisome thoughts about what you should or shouldn't eat, or critical thoughts about your body, you come back with gentleness and precision to what is. This is the technique. And the number of times you can apply it is infinite. With each experience in which your body's intelligence leads you to make choices that feel good in your unique body, you amass evidence for self-trust and self-confidence.

What parts of your Eat to Love path are becoming second nature? When you have experienced slip-ups, how have you responded? In the future, how do you aspire to respond?

When do you experience uncertainty about your choices and thoughts? How have you responded? How do you aspire to respond in the future?

Creating a Sustainable Meditation Practice

In creating a sustainable meditation practice, there are several considerations, including setting realistic expectations, creating enough of a routine that it is more likely to happen, and connecting with the value it brings to your life. It may be tempting when we begin any new behavior to want to do it in an extreme way. In starting a meditation practice, we might vow to meditate an hour every day for the rest of our lives. This is a recipe for disappointment and failure. Such an extreme approach comes from the belief that meditation will fix us, which is not true for two reasons: the first is that you are not broken, and the second is that meditation is not about fixing things but about relating to reality differently.

Relating differently means acknowledging that humans are inherently inconsistent and imperfect beings and that a meditation practice does not have to be extreme to be beneficial. Setting realistic expectations could look like practicing for ten minutes a day, three days a week for a month before re-evaluating and recommitting. Once you feel comfortable and relatively consistent with ten minutes three days a week, you could try five days a week for another month before making any further changes. There is no rush to get anywhere. Allow yourself to be right where you are.

Similar to our thoughts and behaviors around eating and body image, it is what we do with a fair amount of consistency over time that makes the greatest difference in our lives. Having a regular time and place to sit dissolves the barrier of figuring this out day after day. Appending your meditation practice to something you already do, such as meditating right after your morning coffee or tea, increases the likelihood of it happening. Choosing a peaceful and dedicated spot to practice, such as a chair or cushion in a favorite corner of a quiet room, creates a container in which meditation is more likely to occur. Such simple elements of a routine set the stage for sustainability, and compassionately working with the inevitable ups and downs of any long-term change propels us forward. (Several of the resources listed at the back of this book go into greater detail about creating a sustainable meditation practice.)

Acknowledging that change is inherently difficult when beginning a meditation practice is very helpful. Because our practice will be imperfect and at times inconsistent, it is also important to treat ourselves with radical gentleness. Berating ourselves for missing meditation for a day, a week, a month, or even a year is no more productive or motivating than magical eating or hating our bodies was for creating positive change. Self-aggression makes us feel bad about ourselves and less likely to do what makes us feel well. Being gentle and self-compassionate allows us to acknowledge the causes and conditions that led to missing our practice and to take actions that align with our values of working with our minds.

No matter how long or consistent, what really brings us back time and again to our meditation practice is the value it brings to our lives off the cushion. One way to recognize this is to keep a meditation journal. It doesn't have to be anything fancy, just a place to record the date, number of minutes practiced (even if that number is zero), and a word or phrase or few sentences about your practice if you feel so inclined. A meditation journal serves several purposes. It is a record of your meditation practice over time, a repository of your thoughts about your experience both on the cushion and off, a collection of the insights gained as the result of your practice, and an opportunity to observe change and progress over time. It is something for your eyes only. My own experience in keeping a meditation journal is that it helps me be self-compassionate. Keeping track of minutes practiced, whether that be twenty or zero, leads me to be gentle with myself on the days that I don't practice, to let it go and move on to the next day rather than dwelling on any negative feelings. A meditation journal is included in the program available for free download at https://eat2love.com/eat-to-love-at-home-program.

There are other ways to deepen your connection and commitment to your meditation practice. You can get a meditation instructor who has been trained to teach meditation. Practice with others, whether with a virtual or real-life meditation buddy with whom you agree to meditate at the same time, by going to a local meditation center, or by joining a virtual meditation community such at the Open Heart Project Sangha (susanpiver.com). Practicing for longer periods of time, including doing at-home retreats or attending a formal meditation retreat (when you feel ready), does wonders to reinvigorate a meditation practice and to reconnect you with why you started in the first place. Some of the resources available in appendix D offer guidance for deepening your practice.

How would you like to begin your meditation practice? How many minutes? On which days? Where and when? At what point will you come back and re-evaluate?

What do you notice as the result of your practice? How would you like to deepen your connection to your practice?

Our meditation practice is the foundation of and analogy for everything we do on the Eat to Love path. By training our minds and bodies to be present, we reinforce the ability to recognize and work with what is and to show up for ourselves again and again. Zen master, global spiritual leader, poet, and peace activist Thich Nhat Hanh says, "The heart of [meditation] practice is to generate our own presence in such a way that we can touch deeply the life that is here and available in every moment. We have to be here for ourselves; we have to be here for the people we love; we have to be here for life with all its wonders. The message of our [meditation] practice is simple and clear: 'I am here for you.'"

THE PARAMITA

OF WISDOM

THE SIXTH AND final paramita is wisdom, also known as discriminating or clear-seeing knowledge. Wisdom integrates and brings intelligence to the other five paramitas in how we think about food, eating, and our bodies; how we make choices and evaluate them; how we navigate constant change; and how we live our lives and treat our bodies in ways that connect with our values. Wisdom is often stressed in conjunction with compassion and helps us understand the difference between true compassion and idiot compassion, which is enabling harmful habits by taking the path of least resistance. With the paramita of wisdom, we explore how to skillfully balance the outside wisdom of nutrition science with our internal intelligence and set an intention for moving forward on the Eat to Love path.

Graduating from Tufts University with a master's degree in nutrition and having just passed the exam to become a registered dietitian, I ostensibly had the greatest scholarly and scientific knowledge of diet, metabolism, and the body. But I felt like the walking, talking version of Thomas Edison's quote, "We don't know a millionth of one percent about anything." Rather than giving patients diet advice I wasn't convinced of, I decided I was better off on the research and writing side, figuring out who and what to believe in nutrition science.

As a medical writer, I was struck by how challenging it was to conduct high-quality nutrition research because there were so many variables that were impossible to control; how that difficulty affected what we as researchers, clinicians, and consumers knew to be true; and how the resultant nutrition advice seemed to change from one day to the next. As a dieter then myself, I religiously followed the flip-flopping nutrition headlines as if watching a tennis match:

Nuts: Bad. They're like 95 percent fat! Never mind, good: It's healthy fat.

Bread: Bad. Fattening. Good: If it's whole grain! No, bad: Basically legal crack cocaine.

Margarine: Bad. Sad, chemical substitute for butter. No, good: Cheaper and healthier. Nope, bad: Processed food, again.

Butter: Good. Natural, with no trans fats. Nope, bad: Large carbon footprint. Then again, good: Real food, enjoy! But not too much.

Shrimp: Bad. Dangerous harborers of cholesterol. Good: Lean sources of protein! Then again, bad: Possible vehicles for arsenic. And yet, good: What could be wrong with shrimp?

Chocolate: Bad. Fattening and gives you acne. Actually, good: If it's 85 percent dark, it's basically a health food.

Gah! How to keep up? Let alone take it all seriously.

Nearly twenty years later, I now have to look up the individual steps of the Krebs cycle and the nutrient composition of a peanut butter and jelly sandwich, but I feel much wiser. What changed?

While my memory of nutrition science has faded somewhat, I have simultaneously expanded my knowledge, understanding, and practice of living in a constantly changing human body with a mind that either causes great suffering and pain or is curious and feels satisfaction and pleasure. Perhaps the largest part of that has been learning how to place external wisdom in context and always remain open to and aware of my own internal intelligence.

So what is true wisdom?

We tend to associate wisdom with knowledge the mind acquires from books and experts, which influences what we internalize as thoughts and beliefs. External sources of knowledge become what we consider absolute fact. Buddhist philosophy proposes that true wisdom comes from the connection between the mind, heart, and body. We contain basic intelligence that is wise. This does not mean that outside information is useless. Knowledge gained from scientific research, organized exploration, and rigorous experimentation provides valuable insight into how the body and mind work, as well as what foods contribute to health and disease. But outside knowledge should not be mistaken as superior to our own intelligence.

Meditation master Chögyam Trungpa Rinpoche referred to wisdom as "sharpening your intelligence in order to work with yourself." This sharpening process could certainly be likened to the fine-tuning that occurs on the Eat to Love path as our meditation practice and understanding of our bodies and minds deepens, as we learn to stay with our experience regardless of our comfort level, and as we strengthen our ability to recognize and respond to our actual needs.

Our natural intelligence is the awareness that comes from remaining open and attentive in our bodies. This is how the paramita of wisdom is the culmination of the preceding paramitas. It lets us cut through the confusion, distraction, and illusory certainty of magical eating and see things as they are. As we develop the capacity to see things as they are, we realize that some information from books and experts actually can be skillfully incorporated with our innate intelligence. Knowing the difference between useful external information and that which is thinly veiled magical eating makes all of the difference in the full integration of your Eat to Love practice.

Nutrition Wisdom

It's important to begin any section on nutrition with the following facts:

No one food makes you healthy or unhealthy.

No single food or food group causes or prevents disease.

There is no need to detox or cleanse our bodies because our lungs, skin, liver, and kidneys already do this.

Within the confines of what we can control, it is the overall balance of what we eat consistently over a long period of time that has the most profound impact on wellness.

There is a lot we still do not know when it comes to nutrition and health.

Having established that, all foods contain some combination of carbohydrates, protein, and fat—the three macronutrients I described in chapter 3. These macronutrients are broken down differently and are satisfying to the body in different ways, so crafting meals and snacks that combine some carbohydrates, some protein, and some fat is a good practice for meeting the body's needs on many levels. In addition to the macronutrients, our foods contain micronutrients in the form of vitamins and minerals, phytonutrients or plant nutrients, fiber, water, and other compounds that defy easy categorization. What follows should not be considered an exhaustive nutrition reference. Rather, try to look at the information as complementary to your understanding of how various foods *feel* in your body.

Carbohydrates and Fiber

Carbohydrates are the body's primary fuel and the preferred energy for the brain, which needs about 120 grams of glucose (yes, sugar) every day to function optimally. The primary role of carbohydrates is to provide the body with energy. When our bodies get too hungry, such as when we restrict carbohydrates or don't eat consistently, they seek a quick fix, often in the form of sugar or refined carbohydrates, to quickly regulate blood sugar levels and maintain homeostasis or balance. This (coupled with the magical eating belief that we shouldn't have these foods) is why we crave sweets when we aren't adequately fed (which is often in response to the initial avoidance of these foods). Cakes, cookies, candy, pastries, and sweetened beverages meet that immediate energy need but are metabolized so quickly that they don't satisfy us for long and we get hungry again rather soon. This could be confusing.

Carbohydrates that are more slowly broken down by the body are starches or complex carbohydrates, which might also contain fiber. Fiber is found in both soluble and insoluble forms. Soluble fiber, found in oats, barley, beans, peas, carrots, apples, citrus, and psyllium, dissolves in water and helps lower blood cholesterol and blood glucose levels. Insoluble fiber, found in whole-wheat flour, wheat bran, vegetables, beans, and nuts, helps with constipation by moving undigested waste through the intestines. Both complex carbohydrates and fiber help maintain more consistent blood sugar levels, greater satisfaction, and steady energy levels.

In terms of whole foods, carbohydrates are found in whole vegetables and fruits, including sugar cane and sugar beet root; whole grains; rice; beans, which contain protein; and dairy, which contains protein and fat. Carbohydrate-containing processed and packaged foods, meaning those that are derived from the whole foods above, include pasta, breads, crackers, chips, cakes, candy, cookies, pastries, sodas, fruit juices, and energy drinks.

Eating carbohydrates with protein boosts tryptophan, contributing to the production of serotonin and feelings of happiness. Whole grains are important sources of B vitamins. Carbohydrates, including fruits, vegetables, and whole grains, also contain a range of vitamins, minerals, and phytonutrients, which are nutrients with some medicinal value that are found in foods of plant origin.

Protein

Protein is broken down more slowly by the body, which translates into feeling satisfied longer. In addition to providing energy, proteins are responsible for building and repairing muscle tissue. They are involved in the manufacture of hormones, enzymes, and antibodies that allow the body to function and protect it from disease. Protein is found in fish, poultry, meat, eggs, dairy, some dairy substitutes (check the label as some are quite low in protein), beans, tofu, nuts, seeds, vegetables (in small amounts), and protein powders made from whey, soy, rice, pea, or other sources.

Protein-containing foods are also rich sources of vitamins, minerals, and phytonutrients (when from plant sources). When people follow high-protein, low-carbohydrate diets, they often experience bad breath, headaches, and constipation, as well as cravings for sugar and other carbohydrates (exactly what they are restricting). These are not recommended long term (and I recommend them exactly never) because of the potential for damage to the kidneys as the result of metabolizing excess protein. The physical and psychological risks of a very high-protein diet are a good example of how diets are potentially much more dangerous than "can't hurt, right?"

Fat

Fat is the macronutrient that is most slowly broken down by the body, which is why including some fat in your meals and snacks tends to keep you physically satisfied longest. Fat adds a pleasant texture to foods, which might make them more enjoyable. This is why low-fat or fat-free foods tend to be less satisfying, have less staying power, and be less palatable overall. In addition to providing energy, fat is essential for the regulation of sex hormones, the production of neurotransmitters, and the absorption of the fat-soluble vitamins A, D, E, and K. Fats are found in plant foods such as seeds, nuts, olives, coconut, and palm, and in foods of animal origin such as butter, ghee, dairy, meat, and eggs.

There are many different kinds of fats in our foods. Monounsaturated fats and polyunsaturated fats contribute vitamin E and may lower bad (low-density lipoprotein or LDL) blood cholesterol. Monounsaturated fats are found in oils from olives, canola, safflower, and peanut, as well as in avocados, peanut butter, nuts, and seeds. Polyunsaturated fats are found in soybean, corn, and sunflower oil, as well as walnuts, sunflower seeds, soybeans, and other soy products. A special type of polyunsaturated fat is the omega-3 fatty acids, which have strong evidence of a benefit in preventing heart disease, specifically regulating heart rhythm, as well as lowering blood pressure and heart rate, improving the function of blood vessels, decreasing triglyceride levels, and lowering levels of chronic inflammation in the body. (Years ago, when I wrote a book about dietary supplements, one of the few that had the backing of high-quality and reliable scientific studies was omega-3 fatty acids.) Omega-3s are found in fatty fish such as salmon, sardines, and anchovies, as well as in walnuts, flax, hemp, chia, grass-fed meat and dairy products, and some dark green leafy vegetables like spinach and Brussels sprouts.

Saturated fats come primarily from animal sources such as meat, dairy, and eggs. Vegetarian sources of saturated fats include palm and coconut. Saturated fat has been the black sheep of the dietary fat family for a long time for increasing heart disease risk, but more recent evidence suggests that this is not so simple. The association between heart disease risk and saturated fats was drawn from epidemiologic studies that noted a correlation, but that does not mean that saturated fat was the cause. When people cut saturated fat from their diets and increased carbohydrate intake, for example, they *increased* their risk of heart disease. While no one recommends a high-saturated fat diet, there seems to be no reason to cut out sources of saturated fat completely. I would also note that how the source of animal fat is raised and pastured changes the balance of the types of fat, with grass-fed meat and dairy containing generally higher omega-3 levels.

The final kind of fat, trans, is found in small amounts in animal sources but is primarily created through a chemical modification process called hydrogenation, which allows liquid vegetable oils to remain solid at room temperature (such as in margarine). The man-made version of trans fats is cheap, easy to use, and durable, which makes it appealing to food companies. Trans fats increase bad (LDL) and decrease good (HDL, high-density lipoprotein) blood cholesterol and are clearly associated with increased levels of heart disease, stroke, and type 2 diabetes. Trans fats are the only one I advise against consuming. Since a 2013 decision by the U.S. Food and Drug Administration that trans fats are not "generally recognized as safe," their availability has been greatly reduced. If they are present in a food, they are most likely to be labeled as "partially hydrogenated oils" and are listed by name on the nutrition facts label. Trans fats may still be found in some commercially fried foods, packaged baked goods, and margarine-like spreads.

Water

Water, not always thought of in the same class as macro- and micro-nutrients, is truly essential to feeling and being well. Water helps regulate our body temperature, lubricates joints and protects organs and tissues, carries nutrients and oxygen to the cells and makes them readily accessible for metabolism, fights constipation, and helps eliminate waste products from the body. When we aren't getting enough water, it affects our energy levels, sleep, appetite, mood, metabolism, and the functioning of any medications we take. We consume water by drinking it, as well as by eating soups, salads, and fruits and vegetables with high water content.

Probiotics and Prebiotics

The trillions of bacteria that live in your gastrointestinal tract or gut are the focus of a vast field of scientific study. Scientists have discovered there are more bacterial cells in your digestive tract than there are *you* cells in your whole body, which always makes me wonder, *Who are we, really?* Nevertheless, the specific populations, functions, and overall balance of these bacteria may affect our health—including our digestion, immunity, physiology, and even mood—in significant ways. Eating probiotics and prebiotics is one way to improve the balance of gut bacteria and thereby wellness.

Probiotics are the good bacteria in your gut. Some of the most common probiotics include *Lactobacillus* species, *Bifidobacterium* species, *Saccharomyces boulardii*, and *Bacillus coagulans*. Probiotics are found in fermented foods such as yogurt, kefir, kimchi, sauerkraut, miso, kombucha, tempeh, and natto. Prebiotics, on the other hand, serve as food for probiotics; they are the indigestible carbohydrates consumed by probiotics in the digestive tract to compose the various populations of good bacteria in the gut. Sources of prebiotics include whole grains, artichokes, bananas, soybeans, onions, and garlic.

Balancing Nutrition Wisdom with Internal Wisdom

All of the previous nutrition wisdom is wonderful but, as I have emphasized and re-emphasized throughout this exploration of the Eat to Love path, no external source of knowledge should be taken as superior to your own. Or as Chögyam Trungpa Rinpoche put it, "There are enormous problems with thinking that we can only trust in what we were told rather than in how we feel."

As I discussed in earlier chapters, many people fear that giving themselves absolute permission to eat what, when, and how much they truly want to feel satisfied will only lead them to excess. Even if that is initially the response, however, what follows is a normalization of appetites. If at first the pendulum swings from general restriction to unrestrained excess, gradually and with attention and gentleness, that pendulum finds the middle way. I have never worked with someone who did not eventually discover that what her body craved changed from moment to moment, according to different influences, leading her to eat a balanced and varied diet that met her nutrient needs.

Some of the different influences on your appetite include your immediate environment, seasonal changes, cultural heritage, and how well you feel emotionally and physically. If you live in New England, you crave seafood and corn in the summer and hot bowls of creamy clam chowder in the winter. If you take a trip to the Southwest, you seek out good TexMex food. The seasons have a strong effect on the foods you crave, even if some of the basic ingredients remain the same: barbecued ribs and salad, for example, during the summer and hearty beef stew with vegetables in the winter. Despite being in the States for more than ten years, my Sicilian partner craves tomato salads with basil, garlic, and olive oil all summer and can't wait for pasta fagioli, a warm starchy bean and pasta dish, in the winter, demonstrating some seasonal and some cultural influences on his appetite. If you live someplace where the seasons don't bring dramatically different temperatures or where all types of foods are equally available throughout the year, perhaps your tastes are more even-keeled.

How well you feel also strongly influences your desire for certain foods. I often find that feeling ill, particularly if you are dealing with illnesses involving the stomach (or pregnancy), brings your instinctual drives for certain foods to a new level of precision. There is often a stark awareness of what you can and cannot tolerate, or even think about, when you feel nauseated. Being home with a bad cold or flu, on the other hand, is likely to lead you to crave chicken soup, a favorite childhood meal, or whatever other comfort food had significance for you and your family. Other times, you probably crave foods that increase the feel-good chemicals in the brain, such as chocolate, which causes an increase in serotonin, dopamine, and phenylethylamine. All of this is to say that your tastes generally guide you in the direction of meeting your nutritional needs over time.

This isn't a matter of chance. Our bodies are master adapters, hard-wired to survive. How our bodies accumulate and distribute fat is a perfect example. A girl's body-fat makeup is lower until puberty, when it increases to support ovulation and menstruation. As a woman matures, she gains fat first in the breasts, hips, buttocks, and thighs in order to be fertile. A mature ovulating woman's body stores enough energy to survive famine for roughly nine months. During times of famine, about 10 percent of women die, while 50 percent of men do, again suggesting that the human race has survived because of body fat. As a woman's body approaches menopause, her body weight will increase as her metabolism slows, which is associated with a longer lifespan. As hormones shift to menopausal levels, the body increases the generation of fat cells that produce estrogen, many of which accumulate in the abdomen, in order to maintain adequate bone density and to moderate the symptoms associated with menopause. These are just a few examples of the body's intelligence and that it knows what to do. That so many women struggle with the very things that ensure their survival and longevity—bigger hips and thighs in the childbearing years, having belly fat perhaps for the first time upon menopause—is cause for attention, examination, and compassion.

Even in less extreme situations, the body adapts to inconsistent circumstances based on what we eat from day to day, becoming more or less efficient depending on whether we over- or under-consume certain nutrients. We learned earlier how the body adapts to inadequate calories by metabolizing the calories it does receive more sparingly, by becoming efficient, and arming itself to survive. Similarly, if we take in more energy than our body needs to sustain its set point range, for a while it will waste those calories, becoming somewhat less efficient, in order to defend its natural weight. If the body is not taking in enough vitamins and minerals, it will use what it does consume more sparingly. And if it takes in excessive levels of vitamins and minerals, it will eliminate them from the body through the waste products of sweat, breath, urine, and feces (except in the case of fat-soluble vitamins that can cause toxicity, though this is rare). This means that there is absolutely no reason to eat a perfect diet from one day to the next because our bodies adapt to our natural human inconsistency.

Taking this view of our bodies and how they accommodate changes is extremely compassionate. Through feast, famine, injury, healing, illness, recovery, and aging, our bodies are constantly working to protect us.

Bringing Nutrition to Your Personal Eat to Love Path

It is only once you have created a peaceful relationship with food and your body that you should consider bringing nutrition to your Eat to Love path. As with all parts of this process, this should be done with gentleness and a willingness to pay attention to how you respond to the thoughts that arise in your mind and how behavioral changes feel in your body. This always brings to mind the serenity prayer, the saying used during the closure of most twelve-step meetings: "Grant me the serenity to accept the things I cannot change, the courage to change the things I can, and the wisdom to know the difference." In practicing the paramita of wisdom, knowing the difference between what we can change and what we cannot is of paramount importance.

What aspect of your body's wisdom do you most appreciate? What aspect would you like to pay more attention to? In what ways do you have a peaceful relationship with food and your body?

Some underlying concerns my clients express when they wish to integrate nutrition into their Eat to Love path include whether they have obscure food sensitivities and the desire to eat more healthful foods. When clients express concerns about allergies, sensitivities, and intolerances to certain foods, we have a very open and honest conversation about what is contributing to their worries. How much of this is based on media coverage and the latest headlines, cultural fads around avoiding certain foods, generalized hysteria, or actual physical experiences? We also discuss whether their concerns are based on some of the inevitable discomforts in having a human body, such as having gas or feeling tired. We always come back to the fact that, in addition to any validated medical tests that suggest the presence of an allergy, sensitivity, or intolerance, their own bodies are the best indicators of their ability to eat and properly metabolize different foods. We discuss the fact that even if a physical experience is psychosomatic, that is, caused by the belief it will happen, it is still very real.

The way to work with these anxieties is to understand our own beliefs about the food, understand our desire for it, assess our enjoyment of the food, and evaluate the physical effects eating the food has on us. In some cases, people do decide to minimize the amount of certain foods in their diets due to negative physical results. If someone has lactose intolerance, they could decide to cut all dairy from their diet because it is not worth it to them to deal with the consequences of gastrointestinal distress. As a result of this choice, they might encounter sadness or loss. They could choose to experiment with different sources of dairy with varying levels of lactose. Or they could pick and choose when it is worth it to them to have certain foods, such as their favorite ice cream. With very few exceptions, there is no right or wrong choice when it comes to working with potential food sensitivities. Each experience provides information (physical and emotional) on which to base future choices.

What foods do you have concerns about? Where do these concerns likely come from? What is your physical experience of eating this food? What is your emotional experience of eating this food? Going forward, how will you decide whether or how to eat this food?

When clients worry that they are not consuming enough health-promoting foods, I encourage them to focus more on adding in healthful foods rather than taking away anything, which might reawaken the deprivation dragon. As you figure out how to approach this, give yourself permission to forgo the things you don't like; just forget about them. There is no reason to eat Brussels sprouts if you hate them. Focus on what you do enjoy, what feels good in your body, and what contributes to satisfaction and feelings of wellbeing for you. To this end, the following is a list of a few wonderful foods to consider experimenting with:

Whole grains: amaranth, barley, corn, faro, millet, oats, quinoa, rye, sorghum, wheat

Fruits: apples, apricots, bananas, blackberries, blueberries, clementines, cranberries, dates, grapefruit, figs, mango, melon (cantaloupe, Crenshaw, honeydew), nectarines, oranges, papaya, peaches, pineapple, raisins, raspberries, strawberries, tangerines, watermelon

Vegetables: artichokes, avocados, broccoli, broccolini, broccoli rabe, Brussels sprouts, bok choy, cabbage (red and white), carrots (orange, yellow, purple), celery, collard greens, garlic, ginger, kale, kohlrabi, lettuces (red leaf, green leaf, butter, iceberg, arugula, radicchio), onions (white, yellow, red, green), parsnip, peppers (red, green, yellow, orange), potatoes (red skin, Yukon gold, purple), spinach, sweet potatoes, Swiss chard, tomatoes, turnips, zucchini, winter squash (acorn, butternut, spaghetti squash)

Sources of protein: fish, chicken, turkey, beef, lamb, goat, venison, pork, tofu, eggs, cheese, milk, yogurt, nuts, seeds

Sources of omega-3 fatty acids: fatty fish (such as salmon and mackerel), small fish with bones (such as anchovies and sardines), seeds (such as hemp and chia), soybeans, tofu, walnuts

Beans, lentils, and pulses: red lentils, yellow lentils, brown lentils, chickpeas, kidney beans, white beans, cannellini beans, great northern beans, black-eyed peas, peanuts, fava beans

Nuts and seeds: walnuts, cashews, Brazil nuts, hazelnuts, macadamia nuts, pecans, pine nuts, as well as the butters and oils made from these nuts

Fermented foods: miso, kombucha, sauerkraut, pickles, kimchi, kefir, tempeh, natto, yogurt, raw cheeses

Other probiotics and prebiotics: dark chocolate (>70 percent cocoa), green peas, salt-water brined olives, sourdough bread, beet kvass, soft aged cheeses

How will you know when it is the right time to experiment with adding nutrient-rich foods to your diet? Which foods would you like to include? Why? How does it feel to eat them, physically? Emotionally?

When we are ready, the integration of outside knowledge with our own intelligence leads to great satisfaction and feelings of wellness. The willingness to continually consult our bodies, minds, and hearts ensures we are prioritizing our own wisdom on the Eat to Love path.

THE REST OF

YOUR LIFE

YOU MOST LIKELY picked up this book with some goal in mind. Perhaps it was to lose weight, although I hope by now you have abandoned that. Or perhaps it was to change an obsessive and negative relationship with food and your body, which I whole-heartedly support. We all approach new things with objectives and aspirations in mind. That is completely human. At the same time, emphasizing the end point of a particular journey has the effect of taking you out of the moment. The Eat to Love path is as good as any example of this phenomenon. If you were to enter onto this path with your eyes on the end goal, whatever that means for you, you would never fully be able to inhabit your body in a way that might one day lead to your ultimate aspiration. Ah, cruel irony! It is fine to have some hopes in terms of results or outcomes, but when we get too attached to that outcome, we lose the ability to be in the process.

Abandon any hope of fruition

In describing this lojong slogan, many people use the analogy of the archer who understands the dangers of simply focusing on the target. Instead, she must bring awareness to her posture, how the bow is held, and how the arrow is positioned in order to have true aim. The archer is only able to hit the target by being in her body in the moment. Similarly, on the Eat to Love path, our ideas about an outcome get in the way of the experience we are actually having. By projecting into the future, we lose connection with our bodies. Ultimately the focus on any possible outcome is simply a fantasy, an entertaining distraction that has nothing to do with reality, which is the process (not the destination). In his book *The Practice of Lojong: Cultivating Compassion through Training the Mind*, Traleg Kyabgon Rinpoche writes:

> By anticipating the kinds of signs we expect to find, we ensure our continual disappointment because we will think we've failed when those signs don't materialize. All that is really happening is that we can't see the real signs of progress because our preconceived ideas have blinded us to any genuine developments that are taking place. Because our lojong commitment is not about some grand, elaborate fantasy of the future, we should constantly remind ourselves of the futility of hopes and expectations.

Like the paramita of wisdom, this slogan is also a culmination of the previous paramitas. Generosity reminds us to acknowledge and care for the basic needs of our human bodies by attending to our hunger and fullness. Discipline helps us to recognize when we are no longer acting from the position of being inside our bodies and reminds us to continually come back. Patience assures us that progress occurs at its own pace and assists us in speaking to ourselves compassionately. Exertion infuses our every thought, word, and action with the energy and motivation to remain on the path. Meditation solidifies our practice of being in the body, staying with our experience with curiosity and accepting uncertainty, discomfort, and groundlessness. And wisdom supports our ability to discern external knowledge worthy of complementing our internal intelligence. Recognizing that it is how we engage in this process that determines the actual outcome is a form of unconditional love for ourselves.

One element of engaging with this process is our ongoing internal commentary. As we practice being with our experience as it is, our perception has the potential to influence our course, either propelling us forward or causing us to become disheartened.

Be grateful to everyone

Having begun your Eat to Love path, practicing gratitude is a wonderful way to stay afloat as you re-enter the sea of magical eaters. As you have read these pages, done the contemplations, and considered their significance in your life, millions of others have started their next diet or are reeling from the failure of their last one. Being grateful both for what is going well and what continues to be a challenge will orient you to exactly where you are and help you stay on this path.

In Buddhist practice, this slogan often emphasizes being grateful for our obstacles, but I suggest starting with what feels good: recalling the ways in which your basically good body works for you, recognizing the simple pleasure of eating exactly what you want when you want it, and beginning to experience those tiny, spacious gaps in your meditation practice. Once you start paying attention in this way, the list of things for which you are grateful expands exponentially.

Then consider which challenges you could feel gratitude for. There will be no shortage of these on your Eat to Love path, especially when you encounter fat stigma and diet-brainwashed line-toers of all sorts, including an ignorant healthcare system, short-sighted dieting "success stories," and all the members of your circle who haven't changed as you have. As you consider which obstacles could provoke gratitude, observe how they show you your edge, how they reveal something you didn't see before, and how they strengthen your resolve to remain true to yourself. Moving through obstacles genuinely and with gratitude deepens our understanding of and compassion for ourselves and others.

What positive aspects of your Eat to Love path are you grateful for?
What obstacles are you grateful for?

Our human instinct for self-preservation tells us to avoid what feels uncomfortable and lean toward what feels easy. But change doesn't happen without expanding our ability to accommodate, tolerate, and accept discomfort. Turning toward what feels difficult, with gentleness, is what allows us to break through the blocks that keep us stuck in our relationship with food and our bodies. This is because those parts of the process that feel most challenging have something to teach us. Going forward, any time you face a challenge on your Eat to Love path, this final lojong slogan will offer insight into how to greet it.

Train in the three difficulties

Having begun the process of looking at our thoughts and behaviors through the lens of generosity, discipline, patience, exertion, meditation, and wisdom, we likely have a better idea of which parts of the Eat to Love process feel more natural and which ones continue to present challenges. Training in the three difficulties means identifying our challenges and working with them. In order to do this, we need to be very honest with ourselves, figure out where we are, and be willing to meet ourselves there.

The first difficulty is recognizing when we are facing one of our challenges. Without recognition, neuroses arise too quickly for us to really notice and attempt to work with them. As a result, by the time we do notice, we are already hooked and well down the path of damaging habitual reactions. This is fine, and as I mentioned I often refer to this as mindfulness after the fact. But our goal is more and more to train our minds to recognize what is happening in real time. Training in the first difficulty therefore involves slowing things down enough to see ourselves as neuroses arise.

Once we catch ourselves getting hooked, the second difficulty is undermining our neuroses at their root by seeing how they originate with our desire for safety, certainty, and comfort. Whether this means mentally retracing our steps to determine the origin of our particular neurosis or sitting down and mapping out the sequence of events in the past hour, day, and week to identify how energies shifted to culminate in a distorted thought or destructive behavior, this step is about identifying the source of our angst.

The third difficulty is to come back. In this case, it is specifically to return to our bodies in the present moment, to understand what they sense and feel, to continually cultivate self-compassion, and to support ourselves with our meditation practice. We resolve to come back to this again and again whenever we feel ourselves getting hooked.

Train in the three difficulties whenever you find yourself stuck on the Eat to Love path. If you choose to follow the one-week or seven-week program available as a download at https://eat2love.com/eat-to-love-at-home-program, come back to this exercise whenever you find yourself getting hooked, lost, or frustrated.

What challenge do you see yourself facing? What is its root? What allows you to come back to your body? Do you need to rouse generosity, discipline, patience, exertion, meditation, or wisdom?

I have been meditating for nearly a decade now and I still feel like a beginner. Throughout that time, I have attended countless talks and retreats at meditation centers and read many dharma books in my pursuit of wisdom. Like a lot of people, I attend these retreats and read these books to gain something I did not have before: perspective, understanding, and insight. And viewing any topic through the lens of Buddhist teachings never fails to infuse it with a richness that makes me wish I could tattoo the words on the inside of my eyelids. One message is universal: We must rely on our own inherent wisdom and brilliance to live our lives; the dharma is simply a support for this. Whether about romantic love, social injustice, or taking care of our bodies, this pearl remains the same. We could try our best to understand the teachings, but it is up to us to bring compassion, kindness, and open hearts out into the world. Many teachers also have a lovable habit of ending their talks and books with the words "now forget everything." I have always interpreted this advice to mean we should take what made sense to us and leave the rest behind.

Finally, I sincerely appreciate your going on this journey with me. For opening your heart and mind to a new way of relating to your body and contemplating what life could be like if we all trusted in our own basic goodness. Again I would like to acknowledge the many ancient contributing factors that influence how we feel about our selves and shape our relationship with food and our bodies. We are only at the beginning of understanding and learning to address the effects of systemic racism, classism, sexism, sizeism, ableism, ageism, and biases of all varieties. No matter what contributing factors you are working with, it is possible to forever transform your relationship with food and your body. We all deserve to live a life of joy, meaning, confidence, and connection. In fact, it is our birthright.

These are the teachings and practices I use in my own life and the ones I have shared with my clients. There is nothing magical about them and yet they hold within them the potential for discovering the unique wisdom, appetites, and feelings of your body, mind, and heart. Your meditation practice supports you throughout and the paramitas and lojong slogans pave the way for a path that is authentic, dynamic, and ultimately loving.

Only in moving beyond what compelled you to stay compliant will you reach your full potential. I hope that Eat to Love has freed up the mental real estate previously occupied by magical eating so that you can now be authentically yourself. Because the world needs the post–magical eating you. The person who trusts herself, listens to her body, and confidently and skillfully responds to what is needed. The warrior of non-aggression who treats herself with the same gentleness she offers others. The compassionate bodhisattva who will bravely help create the world we are all longing for. Thank you.

Now forget everything.

Appendix A

MINDFUL EATING EXERCISE

MINDFUL EATING EXERCISES are often introduced with a single raisin but, because we are breaking down magical eating beliefs and discovering our true desires, I suggest choosing a food you feel strongly about. Chocolate, gummy worms, pizza, and fries work great. If the first food you think about feels too provocative, choose something less so and gradually work up to more challenging foods.

Begin by sitting down in a peaceful, non-distracting place with your food of choice. Set it in front of you on the table. Before even looking at it, sit up straight and take three mindful and embodied breaths, focusing on how your body feels. Notice any sensations, temperatures, or sense perceptions.

Are you hungry? How hungry? What specific sensations do you feel? How do you know?

Look at the food. Consider all the different individuals who worked to harvest, process, transport, and prepare the food so that it could arrive at this moment.

Notice its color, shape, and texture. What do you observe? What thoughts arise? What do you feel in your body? How are you anticipating eating the food you chose? Happily? Nervously? Fearfully?

Take a piece of the food and place it in the palm of your hand. What is its temperature? What is its weight? What do you feel in your body as you hold the piece of food? Are you salivating? Has your feeling of hunger changed?

Raise the food to your nose and inhale. What does it smell like? Is the smell what you expected? Better, worse, same, or different? How does smelling the food affect your body? Your thoughts?

Hold the food to your lips, just allowing it to rest there. What is it like to touch the food to your body without consuming it immediately? What does your desire for the food feel like?

Place the piece of food in your mouth or bite off a piece. Hold it in your mouth for a moment without moving it. Sense its texture and mass sitting on your tongue. How does it taste?

Now move it around your mouth with your tongue without chewing yet. What do you notice about its texture, temperature, and taste? What changes do you perceive? Has your hunger changed? Has your desire for the food changed?

Begin to chew it slowly. Notice how the texture, taste, and temperature change. Notice the urge to swallow when it first emerges. Continue to chew the food, noticing any changes, until you naturally swallow the food. Notice the residual taste in your mouth. What does your hunger feel like now? What does your desire for the food feel like now? Greater? Lesser?

Repeat the same progression of steps, noticing whether and how the second, third, and fourth bites are different from the first. Notice any changes in taste, hunger, and desire for the food. Notice how you feel about continuing to eat the food. Continue the steps until you decide to stop, and try to be clear about your reason for stopping, knowing there are no right or wrong answers.

Appendix B

TONGLEN MEDITATION

ONGLEN, ALSO KNOWN as "sending and taking," or exchanging self for others, is a special form of meditation practice. Instead of our instinct to keep everything good for ourselves and push away what is painful, or some new-agey approach in which we breathe out the negative and breathe in the positive, in tonglen we breathe in suffering, our own and everyone else's, and breathe out relief from suffering.

When we breathe in the suffering of others, we allow ourselves to fully feel all the unnecessary pain magical eating has wrought. This might feel foreign or scary at first, but it is a very courageous thing to do. The diet culture teaches us to contract, go inward, and think only of ourselves. This practice, on the other hand, invites difficulty with a sense of confidence that we can help bring it to an end. When we practice tonglen, it is with the assurance that we can handle the negativity that we breathe in and that it won't harm us irrevocably; this is how we proclaim our inner strength and goodness. Even though we are focusing on others, tonglen is a very private practice. No one will ever know we are doing it. It is a way to begin turning our energy and attention toward being of benefit to others. Because we are willing to fully feel our pain and the pain of others and to wish them well, tonglen is an intense expression of generosity.

This practice rides the breath just as our awareness rides the breath in shamatha. The breath is always available to us. Any time we see suffering, we can practice tonglen on the spot to acknowledge it and wish for relief of that suffering.

There are four stages to the formal practice. Practice the shamatha technique for five to ten minutes before and after tonglen practice.

1. In the first stage of tonglen, allow your mind to rest in a state of openness, without any specific object.

2. In the second stage of tonglen, begin to work with the texture of what you are sending and taking: breathe in a sense of hot, dark, sticky, and heavy, and breathe out a sense of cool, light, airy relief. Synchronize these with the actual inhale and exhale.

3. In the third stage of tonglen, work with whatever situation feels relevant to you in the moment, bringing to mind some aspect of your Eat to Love path that you are struggling with or the struggles of a specific person.

    Consider the specific details of your own experience. Allow your own challenges with food and body to deepen your compassion for others who also struggle. What part of this journey feels the most painful for you right now as you are reading this? What does your struggle feel like? What might relief of that suffering feel like? Let your own unique experience be how you enter into your tonglen practice.

    When you have a negative feeling about your body, connect with everyone who has ever felt negatively about their bodies, and wish them the ability to accept and love their bodies. Breathe in their and your suffering and breathe out relief.

    When you criticize yourself for some reason, breathe in the pain of everyone who has ever criticized themselves, and breathe out self-compassion.

When you eat in a way that is physically or emotionally uncomfortable, breathe in the suffering of everyone who has ever binged or eaten until sick, and breathe out the confidence to eat according to their body's true needs.

4. In the fourth stage of tonglen, widen the circle, bringing to mind the suffering of all affected by magical eating.

Appendix C

I N LOVING-KINDNESS MEDITATION, we wish safety, happiness, health, and a life marked by ease first for ourselves and progressively for those around us. It is traditionally done by calling to mind our selves first, then a loved one, a neutral person, an enemy, all four (self, loved one, neutral, enemy), and then all beings. Here, we practice loving-kindness a little differently. Instead of different people, we will call to mind different parts of our bodies and wish them well. Because this is difficult, we will alter the order a little bit as well as the specific words we say.

Begin with a few moments of shamatha to settle your mind before beginning this loving-kindness practice. When you are ready, keep your eyes open as in shamatha, or close them if that is more comfortable for you.

Because working with the body is so fraught for many of us, begin by bringing to mind someone or something that is truly easy to love. Perhaps a child or a beloved pet. Once you have that being in mind, say these words silently to yourself:

May you be comfortable
May you be nourished
May you be appreciated
May you be loved

Next, bring to mind a part of your body that you love and find easy to feel positively about. Perhaps it's your eyes, your hands, your nails, or your hair. Bring that body part to mind and say these words silently to yourself:

May you be comfortable
May you be nourished
May you be appreciated
May you be loved

Next, bring to mind a part of your body that is neutral, one that doesn't rouse feelings that are particularly positive or negative. It could be a part of the body you do not think of often, perhaps an internal organ such as your liver, heart, or lungs, or just a body part you take for granted. Say the same words silently to yourself while thinking of this body part:

May you be comfortable
May you be nourished
May you be appreciated
May you be loved

Next, bring to mind a part of your body that feels fraught, something that feels very problematic for you or something you've long fixated on changing. This could be your upper arms, stomach, thighs, or derriere. If the first difficult body part that comes to mind feels too overwhelming, downshift to one that is less so and come back to your original idea when you feel ready. Think of this body part as you say these words silently to yourself:

May you be comfortable
May you be nourished
May you be appreciated
May you be loved

Now bring to mind your whole body, including the positive part, the neutral part, the negative part, and all the other parts that are too many to count. Hold the vision of your whole body in your mind as you say these words to yourself silently:

May you be comfortable
May you be nourished
May you be appreciated
May you be loved

Finally, widen the circle to include all people who have struggled with their bodies and who have dissected them into the parts they like and don't like. Hold the full complement of these people in your mind as you say the words one last time silently to yourself:

May you be comfortable
May you be nourished
May you be appreciated
May you be loved

Close your loving-kindness practice by dropping the words and just noticing whatever feeling or feelings have arisen in your heart, mind, and body. Stay here for several breaths. Finish with a few more minutes of shamatha meditation practice to resettle your mind.

Appendix D

Books

- Linda Bacon and Lucy Aphramor, *Body Respect: What Conventional Health Books Get Wrong, Leave Out, and Just Plain Fail to Understand about Weight* (BenBella, 2014)
- Linda Bacon, *Health at Every Size: The Surprising Truth about Your Weight* (BenBella, 2010)
- Pema Chödrön, *Taking the Leap: Freeing Ourselves from Old Habits and Fears* (Shambhala, 2010)
- Pema Chödrön, *The Places That Scare You: A Guide to Fearlessness in Difficult Times* (Shambhala, 2002)
- Pema Chödrön, *When Things Fall Apart: Heart Advice for Difficult Times* (Shambhala, 2000)
- Jan Chozen Bays, *Mindful Eating: A Guide to Rediscovering a Healthy and Joyful Relationship with Food* (Shambhala, 2017)
- Rick Hanson, *Buddha's Brain: The Practical Neuroscience of Happiness, Love and Wisdom* (New Harbinger, 2009)
- Caroline Knapp, *Appetites* (Counterpoint, 2011)
- Traleg Kyabgon, *The Practice of Lojong: Cultivating Compassion through Training the Mind* (Shambhala, 2007)

- Judith Matz and Ellen Frankel, *Beyond a Shadow of a Diet: The Comprehensive Guide to Treating Binge Eating Disorder, Compulsive Eating, and Emotional Overeating* (Routledge, 2014)
- Judith Matz and Ellen Frankel, *The Diet Survivor's Handbook: 60 Lessons in Eating, Acceptance and Self-Care* (Sourcebooks, 2006)
- Kristin Neff, *Self-Compassion: The Proven Power of Being Kind to Yourself* (William Morrow, 2011)
- Susan Piver, *Start Here Now: An Open-Hearted Guide to the Path and Practice of Meditation* (Shambhala, 2015)
- Rebecca Scritchfield, *Body Kindness: Transform Your Health from the Inside Out—And Never Say Diet Again* (Workman, 2016)
- Jessamyn Stanley, *Every Body Yoga: Let Go of the Fear, Get on the Mat, Love Your Body* (Workman, 2017)
- Shunryu Suzuki and Trudy Dixon, *Zen Mind, Beginner's Mind: Informal Talks on Zen Meditation and Practice* (Shambhala, 2011)
- Evelyn Tribole and Elyse Resch, *Intuitive Eating: A Revolutionary Program That Works* (St. Martin's Griffin, 2012)
- Evelyn Tribole and Elyse Resch, *The Intuitive Eating Workbook* (New Harbinger, 2017)
- Chögyam Trungpa, *Shambhala: The Sacred Path of the Warrior* (Shambhala, 2007)
- Lindy West, *Shrill* (Hachette, 2016)

Websites and Blogs

- Association for Size Diversity and Health (sizediversityandhealth.org)
- Be Nourished (benourished.org)
- The Body Is Not an Apology (thebodyisnotanapology.com)
- The Body Positive (thebodypositive.org)
- The Center for Mindful Eating (thecenterformindfuleating.org)
- Dances with Fat (danceswithfat.wordpress.com)
- Green Mountain at Fox Run (fitwoman.com/blog)
- Health at Every Size Community (haescommunity.com)

- Intuitive Eating (intuitiveeating.org)
- Isabel Foxen Duke (isabelfoxenduke.com)
- Kristin Neff (self-compassion.org)
- The Militant Baker (themilitantbaker.com)
- Virgie Tovar (virgietovar.com/blog)

Podcasts and More

- The Body Kindness Podcast with Rebecca Scritchfield, RDN (bodykindnessbook.com/podcast/)
- The BodyLove Project (jessihaggerty.com/blppodcast)
- Dietitians Unplugged (dietitiansunplugged.libsyn.com)
- Food Psych (christyharrison.com/foodpsych)
- Intuitive Eating online community and Chat with an Intuitive Eating Pro series (free to sign up, intuitiveeatingcommunity.org)
- Love, Food (juliedillonrd.com/lovefoodpodcast)
- Nutrition Matters (paigesmathersrd.com/podcast)
- Recovery Warriors (recoverywarriors.com/podcast)

Eating Disorder Support

- Academy for Eating Disorders (aedweb.org)
- Binge Eating Disorder Association (bedaonline.com)
- Eating Disorder Hope (eatingdisorderhope.com)
- EDReferral.com
- National Eating Disorders Association (nationaleatingdisorders.org)

Note: a handful of books and resources in this list might not be perfectly aligned with the Eat to Love view in that they contain subtle weight stigma or promotion of magical eating. They are included as an attempt to enrich your practice and to *not* throw out the baby with the bathwater. I trust your judgment.

Acknowledgments

O MY BELOVED friend, colleague, and meditation instructor, Susan Piver. Your wisdom, humor, commitment, practice, and path inspire me to show up authentically every day. Thank you for seeing something in me I did not. I love you beyond words.

To my dharma teachers, Chögyam Trungpa, Pema Chödrön, Jan Chozen Bays, and Sarah Napthali. Thank you for devoting your lives to our benefit. Your teachings have given me a life worth living.

To my personal and professional inspirations, Evelyn Tribole, Elyse Resch, Deb Burgard, Linda Bacon, Tracy Tylka, Marsha Hudnall, Megrette Fletcher, Chevese Turner, Caroline Knapp, Roxane Gay, RuPaul Charles, Sonya Renee Taylor, Virgie Tovar, Emme, Lindy West, and Jessamyn Stanley. You are the true warrior bodhisattvas. Without your work, there would be nothing to view through the lens of the dharma.

Thank you, Crystal Gandrud, for not only expertly editing this manuscript but also for living it. Your excellence, discernment, and exquisite presence provided me the confidence and exertion I needed to complete this offering. It is as much yours as it is mine.

To Lisa Fehl. Thank you for your unwavering support, creativity, and encouragement. Your magic works wonders, Angel Witch.

To the Open Heart Project Mommy Sangha of momtrepreneurs, mommysattvas, and crazy wisdom compassion masters. Thank Buddha for you.

To my professional sangha, Mary Jane Detroyer, Monika Saigal, Robin Millet, Justine Roth, and Alexis Conason: your humor, wisdom, and commitment keep me sane. Thank you.

Thank you to Page Two strategies for your wisdom, expert guidance, and for being as excited about this book as I am.

To Colleen Lutz Clemens, Sean Michael McCormick, Tracy Lessor, Jennifer Eliasi Teich, Maureen Gill, and Jordan Hayles. Thank you for being the friends I can pick up with as if not a day has passed.

To Giovanna Cinquemani, for all those extra babysitting hours while I worked on this manuscript. Thank you for loving our little person. You are part of our family now.

To Richie Mastascusa, for guiding and strengthening my body through pregnancy, post-pregnancy, and recovery from spinal surgery. And for bringing my music knowledge into the new millennium. Werk!

To my family. My mom, Terry Hollenstein: thank you for giving me life, a love of food, ten thousand encouraging cards along the way, and always wanting the best for me. And for trusting me to share some of our dirty dieting laundry. May we all overcome. My dad, Peter Hollenstein: thank you for being the person who cries at movies and begins learning Italian in your seventies. You are an artist and a truly gentle soul. My sister, Melissa Hollenstein Thibault, and brother in law, Jonathan Thibault: thank you for your humor and for always being there, no matter what.

To Domenico Peter Ventura. My Mimmo. I started this book when you were in my belly. Thank you for reminding me of the brilliance we are born with. Your curiosity, sensitivity, humor, and joy surprise and delight me on the daily. You are my favorite person.

And to my domestic(ated) partner, Andrea Ventura. Thank you for supporting me on this journey even when you didn't totally understand it. You are the friend, partner, lover, and father to our child that I always dreamed of. *Ti voglio tanto bene.*

About the Author

J ENNA HOLLENSTEIN, MS, RD, is a registered dietitian, non-diet nutrition therapist, and meditation instructor with a private practice in Manhattan, where she works with people struggling with chronic dieting, disordered eating, and eating disorders. Jenna is passionate about helping people transcend the diet culture, rediscover the pleasures of eating and being in their bodies, and live life with joy, connection, and compassion. Jenna is also the author of *Understanding Dietary Supplements* and the memoir *Drinking to Distraction*. To learn more about Jenna's work and to download the Eat to Love at-home program, please visit https://eat2love.com/eat-to-love-at-home-program.

Made in United States
North Haven, CT
21 October 2021

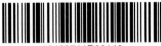